All about Your Eyes

SHARON FEKRAT, M.D., FACS, AND

JENNIFER S. WEIZER, M.D., EDITORS

FOREWORD BY PAUL LEE, M.D., J.D.

ILLUSTRATIONS BY STANLEY M. COFFMAN

Duke University Press   Durham and London   2006

© 2006 Duke University Press
All rights reserved
Printed in the United States of
America on acid-free paper ∞
Designed by CH Westmoreland
Typeset in Minion by Tseng
Information Systems, Inc.
Library of Congress Cataloging-
in-Publication Data appear on
the last printed page of this
book.

Contents

6 · Conjunctiva and Sclera

7 · The Cornea

8 · The Lens

9 · Retina and Choroid

Illustrations

Foreword

PAUL LEE, M.D., J.D.

Amid the tumultuous changes in today's health care system, patients are often challenged to understand and participate effectively in their own care. Worries about insurance coverage, co-payments and deductibles, and other financial concerns often detract from a patient's ability to navigate the care system and work with his or her physician to obtain the best care available. It is not surprising to learn that older patients often have the most difficulty successfully utilizing the full range of available health care services.

For patients with eye diseases, this is of special concern. The likelihood of suffering from a major chronic eye disease rises with age and increases dramatically after the age of sixty-five. Indeed, nearly half of Medicare beneficiaries will have glaucoma, macular degeneration, diabetic retinopathy, or a combination of these conditions over the next few years. When we include cataract and associated conditions, it is clear that nearly every older American will at some point have to deal with eye conditions that could reduce his or her vision.

At the same time, increasing demands for care, and the resulting pressures on health care providers to see more patients, may mean that time for education and counseling will become increasingly precious. When the first wave of Baby Boomers reaches Medicare age in 2011, these forces may combine to create a "perfect storm" within our health care system. Because Baby Boomers are more likely to demand detailed information and to be more skeptical than past generations, physicians and other providers will be hard pressed to meet the needs of this growing number of patients, let alone more intense demands from each patient.

The signs of these forthcoming changes—and fortunately the solutions to these challenges—have been with us for quite a while.

Pioneers have pointed out the importance of "patient-centered care" and "integrative medicine." Medical information accounts for one of the largest uses of the internet in the United States. Medical reporters are celebrities and household names. In studies of patients' expectations, patients tell us that they want a competent physician who will talk to them.

It is in meeting this growing (and soon to be exploding) need that this book is so valuable. Drs. Sharon Fekrat and Jennifer Weizer have organized an important and highly useful volume designed to help those interested in eye health and eye diseases to better understand and participate in their own eye care. As such, the book provides critical information to a population often lacking in it and extends the ability of some of our country's best eye doctors to reach patients, their families, and other interested readers in the United States and throughout the world.

The early chapters present a basic background on the eye and vision. The book proceeds to discuss common refractive vision problems that affect most people and then highlights those eye conditions identified as most important by the National Eye Institute and the World Health Organization. Where appropriate, the book teaches by specific disease; in other instances, it adopts a more generic approach to syndromes or presenting symptoms.

Readers will learn much about the most common and important eye conditions. But more importantly, this book demystifies eye diseases and will help patients and their families deal with visual impairment in the event that interventions are unsuccessful. By helping readers better understand and participate in their care, *All about Your Eyes* will help empower patients and those who care about them to better navigate the oncoming storms in our health care delivery system.

Introduction

JENNIFER S. WEIZER, M.D. · SHARON FEKRAT, M.D.

We came up with the idea for this book when we realized that our eye patients needed a reliable, easy-to-understand guide to eye care. Often in the eye doctor's office, the eye seems like a mysterious organ, and the unfamiliar words used to describe the eye and eye diseases can be difficult to understand. We have designed this reference text as a guide to the eyes and how they work, what can go wrong with them, and what to do about it.

Our first few chapters demystify the structure and function of the eyes, the eye exam, and what to expect from your eye doctor. We then describe various eye diseases, including common problems such as cataract, glaucoma, age-related macular degeneration, and diabetic retinopathy that affect a large part of the population. We also include chapters on up-to-date surgical techniques for eye problems, as well as chapters on refractive and cosmetic eye surgery. We have listed noncommercial websites for each chapter so that you may further explore the topics in this book. Because the book is intended for the nonmedical reader, it is written in easy-to-understand language and includes a glossary of technical terms.

All about Your Eyes is intended not only for patients with eye diseases but for their family members, who can read it to gain an understanding of what their loved ones are experiencing. This book can also help people without known eye problems by explaining how healthy eyes work and describing the symptoms of eye diseases, so that they may perhaps be diagnosed sooner.

Although reading about your eyes can provide a useful understanding of the subject, this book is not designed as a substitute for seeing your eye doctor: medicine is far from a cookbook science. Only you and your eye doctor together can devise an individual approach that works best for you and your eyes.

All about Your Eyes

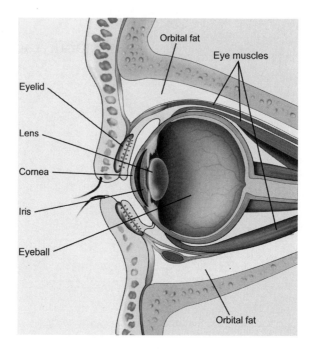

Orbital fat

Eye muscles

Eyelid

Lens

Cornea

Iris

Eyeball

Orbital fat

1 Side view of the eyeball behind the eyelids.

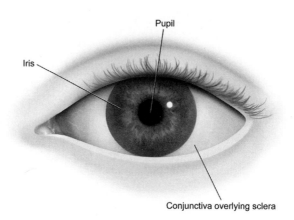

Pupil

Iris

Conjunctiva overlying sclera

2 Front view of the eyeball.

1 · Anatomy of the Eye and How It Works

Eyelids

RAVI CHANDRASHEKHAR, M.D., MSEE

The eyelids act as a protective covering for the eyeball while helping to keep its surface lubricated. Eyelashes help trap debris and prevent unwanted materials from entering the eye, and the lids themselves block excess light and foreign objects. The eyelids distribute the tear film evenly during blinking, and tiny glands on the edges of the eyelids produce oil which slows evaporation of the tear film and helps lubricate the eye's surface.

The eyelids are composed of several layers. The outermost layer is the skin, followed by a layer of muscle and more supportive tissue and finally by the innermost conjunctiva. The eyelid muscles help open and close the eyelids while giving them tone and shape. The conjunctiva on the inside of the eyelids is continuous with the conjunctiva on the surface of the eyeball.

Conjunctiva

RAVI CHANDRASHEKHAR, M.D., MSEE

The conjunctiva is a thin, transparent mucous membrane that covers three parts of the eye. It lines the inner surfaces of the upper and lower eyelids. It helps form a barrier inside the eyelids that separates the front half of the eyeball from the back half (this space is called the fornix). Finally, the conjunctiva becomes even thinner and continues over the front surface of the eyeball up to the edge of the cornea known as the limbus.

The conjunctiva serves as the outer protective surface of the eyeball, and the conjunctiva that lines the eyelids provides a smooth interface with the conjunctiva on the surface of the eyeball to make blinking and eye movements comfortable. Blood vessels in the conjunctiva help nourish the eye as well.

Although the conjunctiva is normally transparent, blood or inflammation can cause it to appear red or pink (as in subconjunctival hemorrhage or conjunctivitis).

Sclera

RAVI CHANDRASHEKHAR, M.D., MSEE

The sclera is the tough, white, outer layer of the eyeball. It begins at the edge of the cornea, or limbus, and surrounds the eyeball until it reaches the optic nerve in the back of the eye. The whiteness of the sclera gives the eye its white appearance outside the cornea, although the sclera is covered with clear conjunctiva in the front of the eye. In the back of the eye, the sclera lies just outside the choroid layer. The sclera is made of tightly woven interlocking fibers which protect the eyeball from injury and help it to hold its spherical shape.

Eye movement is controlled by six muscles that attach at various locations on the sclera. By pulling on the sclera, the muscles cause the eye to move in the desired direction. The sclera also contains tiny blood vessels which provide its nourishment.

Cornea

RAVI CHANDRASHEKHAR, M.D., MSEE

The cornea is the clear, round, central window in the front of the eyeball which light travels through to enter the eye. It is made up of five curved, transparent tissue layers and measures about 12 millimeters in diameter. Unlike other parts of the eye the cornea does not have a blood supply, but it does contain tiny nerves which make the cornea very sensitive to pain when touched or scratched.

The purposes of the cornea include protecting the eye, allowing light to enter the eye (hence the cornea is clear), and bending and refracting the light so that images can focus on the retina and travel to the brain, allowing us to see. Alterations in the normal, curved shape of the cornea can cause astigmatism, and changes in the cornea's shape also contribute to nearsightedness and far-sightedness.

Iris

RAVI CHANDRASHEKHAR, M.D., MSEE

The iris is the colored, circular part of the eye that forms the pupil in its center. Irises range in color from blue to green to brown, depending on how much melanin, or pigment, they contain. A person with a brown iris has more melanin-containing cells in the iris than a person with a blue iris.

The iris divides the front part of the eye into two chambers. Eye structures in front of the iris are part of the anterior chamber, while structures behind the iris are part of the posterior chamber. The iris itself is made of muscles and tissues that adjust the size of the pupil so that the appropriate amount of light can travel though the pupil to form an image on the retina. This mechanism is similar to that of a camera, in which the amount of light to which the film is exposed is determined by the aperture of the lens.

The iris contains two sets of muscles. One set of muscles dilates the pupil so that more light can pass through to the retina. The other set of muscles constricts the pupil to let less light through. The body's central nervous system controls these muscle systems to let in the appropriate amount of light.

At the outer edge of the iris is the ciliary body, which is composed of iris-like tissue. The zonules that support the lens insert into the ciliary body for support. The ciliary body contains muscles which contract and relax as the lens accommodates for near vision.

Pupil

RAVI CHANDRASHEKHAR, M.D., MSEE

The pupil is not an actual physical structure; rather, it is defined as the dark-appearing round space in the middle of the iris. Light passes through the pupil to reach the retina and form an image. Iris muscles control the size and shape of the pupil so that the proper amount of light reaches the retina. A larger pupil lets more light pass through the eye, which is useful in dim light, while a smaller pupil lets less light reach the retina, such as in bright sunlight.

The average diameter of the pupil is approximately 3 millimeters. Because the size of the pupil is regulated by the brain, checking the pupils' reaction to light is a basic test of brain function.

Chambers

RAVI CHANDRASHEKHAR, M.D., MSEE

The space inside the front part of the eyeball is divided into two main areas, or chambers. The front, or anterior, chamber is the space between the cornea and the front of the iris. The back, or posterior, chamber is between the back of the iris and the front of the vitreous gel. The posterior chamber surrounds the front of the lens.

The anterior chamber is filled with aqueous humor, a clear fluid produced by the eye to nourish itself. The aqueous humor normally drains out through the anterior chamber angle, which is at the edges of where the cornea meets the iris. This balance between production and drainage of aqueous humor helps to maintain healthy eye pressure.

Lens

RAVI CHANDRASHEKHAR, M.D., MSEE

The purpose of the lens is to refract, or bend, light so that an image can form on the retina for the brain to "see." The cornea performs about 70% of the necessary bending of light rays, while the lens performs the other 30%. The lens is shaped like a lentil and is located behind the iris, where it is suspended in its own clear capsular bag by fibers called zonules. The lens is made of proteins that form a crystal-like structure, resulting in a clear lens that allows light to pass through it. As a person ages, the proteins in the lens continue to grow, which makes the lens larger, more cloudy, and yellowish-brown. This normal aging is called a cataract.

When a person looks at an object up close, the zonules change their tension on the lens, causing it to change its shape slightly. This response is called accommodation. As the lens ages and becomes thicker, it cannot change its shape as easily, and near objects become more difficult to focus on without the help of reading glasses.

Vitreous

RAVI CHANDRASHEKHAR, M.D., MSEE

The vitreous, or vitreous humor, is a transparent, gel-like substance in the vitreous cavity in the back of the eyeball. The vitreous occupies about 80% of the volume of the eyeball and helps the eye to maintain its spherical shape. The vitreous is composed of 99% water and 1% protein. It is attached to the retina at several points.

The vitreous gel becomes more liquid as a person ages. As it liquefies, the vitreous moves more freely inside the eye and its attachments to the retina can break free. This causes a posterior vitreous detachment, which is a normal aging change but can also occasionally lead to a retinal break or retinal detachment. The loose vitreous gel that moves inside the eye can cause floaters.

Retina

RAVI CHANDRASHEKHAR, M.D., MSEE

The retina is a thin layer of complex nerve tissue that lines the inside back wall of the eyeball. It is located between the vitreous and the choroid. The front edge of the retina is located at the ora serrata, just behind the ciliary body, and the back edge is at the border of the optic nerve. The retina contains its own blood vessels to provide itself with nutrients and oxygen. The small central area of the retina which is responsible for detailed central vision is called the macula.

The retina is composed of ten cell layers, all of which work together to receive images made of light rays, transfer those images into electrical signals, and send the signals to the brain to be "seen." Two types of specialized retinal cells, called rod and cone photoreceptors, play an especially important role in this visual process. These rods and cones actually change the incoming light rays from a visual image into electrical signals. The rods process black-and-white vision, while the cones process color vision. The electrical signals they produce travel through specialized nerve cells in the retina, which all come together to form the optic nerve. Because the macula is responsible for detailed color vision, there are more cone photoreceptors here than in the surrounding, or peripheral, retina.

Retinal Pigment Epithelium and Bruch's Membrane

RAVI CHANDRASHEKHAR, M.D., MSEE

Two important tissue layers that line the inside of the eyeball separate the retina from the choroid. The retinal pigment epithelium lies directly beneath the retina. It is made of a single layer of cells that provide nutrients to the overlying rod and cone photoreceptors in the retina and keep them functioning properly. Under the retinal pigment epithelium is Bruch's membrane. The purpose of this tissue layer is to separate the retina and retinal pigment epithelium from the choroid underneath. Because the choroid contains its own specialized blood vessels, Bruch's membrane keeps these vessels separated from the retina to allow it to function normally. In age-related macular degeneration, for example, cracks in Bruch's membrane occur, allowing choroidal vessels to grow underneath the retina and cause vision loss.

Choroid

RAVI CHANDRASHEKHAR, M.D., MSEE

The choroid is a layer of pigmented vascular tissue found between the retina and the sclera. It contains many blood vessels which supply the eye and retina with necessary nutrients and oxygen. The choroid, ciliary body, and iris together are known collectively as the uvea, since they are all connected and composed of similar tissue. Besides containing blood vessels for the eye, the uvea is pigmented to absorb excess light as it enters the eye.

Optic Nerve

RAVI CHANDRASHEKHAR, M.D., MSEE

The optic nerve carries electrical signals from the retina toward the part of the brain known as the visual cortex. Nerve fibers from the retina come together in a bundle to form the optic nerve, which is connected to the brain. The fibers run through the brain, eventually reaching the back area, where the visual cortex is located.

The optic nerve contains the central retinal artery and central retinal vein that run to and from the eyeball to provide much of its blood supply and return. The optic nerve is surrounded by the same layers of tissue that surround the rest of the brain, making the optic nerve truly part of the brain. The back end of the optic nerve connects to the optic chiasm in the brain, which is a structure where both optic nerves (one from each eye) are joined.

The front end of the optic nerve, which is at the back of the eyeball, can be seen during a dilated eye examination. Your eye doctor examines the optic nerve here to look for signs of glaucoma, optic nerve swelling, or other optic nerve diseases.

The optic nerve can be thought of as the cable that carries information from the eye to the brain, where that information can be processed into an image that is "seen." Any damage to the optic nerve can disrupt this flow of information and lead to vision problems. Damage to the optic nerve can be permanent. A neuro-ophthalmologist specializes in diseases of the optic nerve.

Orbit

RAVI CHANDRASHEKHAR, M.D., MSEE

The eyeball sits in a cavity in the head known as the orbit, or eye socket. The orbit is shaped like a pyramid with four walls lying on its side, its tip pointed toward the brain. The walls of the orbit are made of seven bones which protect the eyeball from injury, and much of the orbit behind the eyeball is filled with fat to provide a supportive cushion for the eye. Also in the orbit are blood vessels, eye muscles which move the eyeball, the lacrimal gland which produces tears to lubricate the eye, and nerves involved in vision, sensation, and eye movements.

At the back of the orbit is a small opening known as the optic canal, through which the optic nerve passes on its way to the brain. Other blood vessels and nerves connected to the brain also enter the orbit through this opening.

Pathways from the Eye to the Brain

RAVI CHANDRASHEKHAR, M.D., MSEE

In order for us to see, light must travel through the eye all the way back to the brain, where it is processed so we can "see" an image. First, light rays strike the cornea, where they are bent, or refracted. These light rays then pass through the anterior chamber and the pupil. Next they reach the lens, where they are refracted even further. The light then passes through the clear vitreous and hits the retina in the back of the eye, where light is converted into electrical signals. These electrical signals travel through the optic nerve to the optic chiasm, where the information from both eyes is combined.

In the brain the optic chiasm splits into two pathways known as the optic tracts, one on each side of the brain. The optic tracts continue to travel back toward the visual cortex of the brain, spreading out into the optic radiations. These optic radiations finally reach the visual cortex at the back of the head, where the brain processes the electrical signals into images. With so many nerve fibers traveling through the brain, a large part of the brain's area is involved in

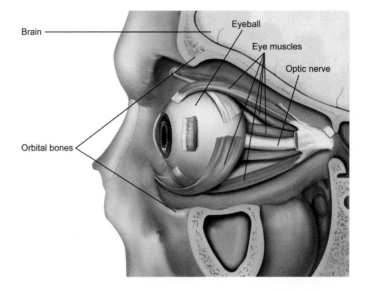

3 The eyeball sits in the orbit and has eye muscles attached to it.

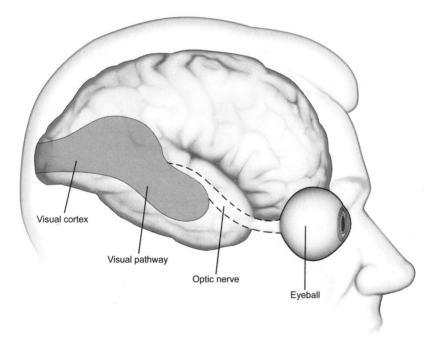

4 The visual pathway connects the eyeballs to the brain.

the visual system. Any disruption anywhere along the visual pathway can lead to vision loss.

http://www.stlukeseye.com/Anatomy.asp
http://www.eyemdlink.com/anatomy.asp

How the Eye Works

CAROL J. ZIEL, M.D.

As you can see by reading about the anatomy of the eye, there are many structures that are necessary to give us vision. The human visual system is designed to give us depth perception, which means that we can tell which objects are in front of or behind other objects. Depth perception is useful for doing simple tasks, such as pouring a cup of coffee or driving a car, and is even more important in tasks that require detailed eye-hand coordination, such as performing surgery.

How exactly are the eyes designed to give us depth perception? First, both eyes must have normal or near normal vision to work together. Glasses or contact lenses may be needed to obtain normal, or 20/20, vision. Then, the eyes must be aligned in the skull so that they are facing in the same direction and are close enough together that each eye's peripheral vision, or side vision, overlaps considerably with that of the other. If we cover one eye and then the other when looking at an object, we can tell that each eye is seeing the same object just a little differently. As we cover and uncover each eye, it is as if the object moves a little to the right or to the left. Therefore, each eye receives a slightly different image that is sent to the brain for processing.

The ability of the brain to process or blend these two similar images is called fusion. The brain must be able to maintain the blending of these images into one image as the eyes move together in various directions. High-level fusion develops completely during childhood, usually between the ages of 5 and 9.

http://mercyhealthpartners.client.web-health.com/web-health/topics/
GeneralHealth/generalhealthsub/generalhealth/eye/
how_eye_work.html

2 · Preventive Eye Care

Recommended Schedule for Eye Exams

CAROL J. ZIEL, M.D.

Eye exams are recommended throughout life to ensure the proper development and maintenance of good vision. These exams allow the eye doctor to discover any problems that can be corrected to prevent or reverse vision loss.

Vision screenings are performed on newborns and babies by eye doctors or pediatricians to ensure that there are no obstructions in the visual pathway (such as congenital cataracts), that the eyes are looking straight ahead and are aligned together, and that each eye is seeing well independently. Vision screenings should be performed every two years unless problems arise sooner. At the age of 5 or when the child begins school, a formal eye exam is recommended so that the visual acuity, or level of vision, can be measured accurately.

Once the vision has developed completely in adults, a full eye exam every ten years between the ages of 20 and 39 may be sufficient unless a patient has a known eye problem or risk factors for eye disease. During those years, eye evaluations for glasses or contact lenses may be necessary. After 40 to 45 years of age, a full, comprehensive eye exam, including dilation, should be done every two years to check for eye problems such as glaucoma, age-related macular degeneration, and cataract, as these diseases increase with age. People with known eye problems may need to be examined more often. Patients with diabetes should be examined at least yearly and sometimes more often, depending on the degree of diabetic eye disease.

http://www.aao.org http://www.opted.org http://www.aoa.org
http://www.oaa.org

Eye Care Specialists: Opticians, Optometrists, and Eye M.D.'s (Ophthalmologists)

CAROL J. ZIEL, M.D.

Opticians · Opticians are professionals who fit and dispense corrective eyewear including glasses, contact lenses, low-vision aids, and ocular prostheses (artificial eyes). To become an optician, one must complete several years as an apprentice or attend a college program that teaches the skills necessary to fit corrective eyewear. After this training opticians can apply to become licensed or certified, depending on the requirements of the state where they practice.

Optometrists · The American Optometric Association defines a doctor of optometry (O.D.) as "an independent primary health care provider who examines, diagnoses, treats and manages diseases and disorders of the visual system, the eye and associated structures." Services provided by optometrists include prescribing glasses and contact lenses, rehabilitating the visually impaired, and diagnosing and treating selected ocular diseases. Optometrists do not attend medical school. They do not perform surgery and usually do not perform laser treatments. Doctors of optometry must successfully complete a four-year accredited degree program at a school or college of optometry. Optometrists must be licensed by the state in which they practice.

Eye M.D.'s (Ophthalmologists) · Ophthalmology is a branch of medicine specializing in the anatomy, function, diseases, and surgical treatment of the eye. An eye M.D., or ophthalmologist, is a medical doctor (that is, an M.D., or occasionally a D.O., who has attended osteopathic school) specially trained to provide the full spectrum of eye care, from prescribing glasses and contact lenses to complex and delicate eye surgery. Many eye M.D.'s are also involved in scientific research about the causes and cures of vision problems and eye diseases. After four years of medical school and one year of internship, every eye M.D. spends a minimum of three years in ophthalmology residency (hospital-based training). Often an eye M.D. spends an additional one to two years training in a subspecialty, or specific area, of eye care (such as glaucoma, retina, oculoplastics, neuro-ophthalmology, cornea and refractive ophthalmology, or pediatric ophthalmology). Almost all eye M.D.'s are board-certified. A board-certified eye M.D. has passed a rigorous two-part examination given by the American Board of Ophthalmology and designed to assess his or her knowledge, experience, and skills. Like all M.D.'s, ophthalmologists must be licensed in the state in which they practice.

http://www.aao.org/aao/about/eyemds.cfm
http://www.aoa.org/eweb/DynamicPage.aspx?site=
    AOAstage&WebCode=DoctorofOpt
http://www.oaa.org/navbar/1consumer/index.asp

The Eye Exam

CAROL J. ZIEL, M.D.

The goals for eye exams in children and adults are somewhat different. With children it is important to ensure the full development of normal binocular vision, in which both eyes work together to perceive depth. With adults the goal of the eye exam is to maximize the visual potential that each person has developed in childhood, and to maintain that vision throughout his or her lifetime. Many components of the eye exam are nonetheless the same for all ages.

For all ages, the first part of the eye exam is to take a history. The eye doctor or eye technician asks the patient if he or she has any vision problems and if so, whether anything makes these problems better or worse. For example, does the patient wear glasses or contact lenses? Has he or she had any eye diseases, eye surgeries, or eye injuries in the past? Reviewing a patient's family history of eye diseases, such as glaucoma, diabetes, and age-related macular degeneration, can help the eye practitioner focus on each patient individually, so that all potential eye problems are addressed. Also, reviewing the patient's other medical problems and medications helps to assess related health problems.

The comprehensive eye exam assesses the functional as well as the anatomic status of each eye. After the history, the next task in the eye exam is to test the visual acuity, or level of vision, in each eye. Using one eye at a time, the patient reads the eye chart, sometimes at more than one distance and often wearing glasses or contact lenses. If the vision is less than 20/20, a refraction is performed either manually or with a machine to determine what the visual potential would be if the refractive error were corrected. This refraction tests whether a patient's visual acuity could be improved by changing his or her glasses prescription. Eye alignment and motility are tested to ensure that that both eyes are lined up together and that they move together in all directions. The pupils are checked to make sure that the two are equal and that they respond normally to light. Eye pressure is measured, using one of several methods. Each eye's visual field, or peripheral vision, is checked. The external appearance of the eyes and eyelids is noted to make sure that they are properly positioned and that the eyes can open and close normally.

The eye doctor then examines each eye with a slit lamp, starting with the front of the eye and moving toward the back. The slit lamp is a modified microscope that magnifies the eye. The eyelids, eyelashes, conjunctiva, sclera, cornea, iris, and anterior chamber are examined for any abnormalities. Then the pupils can be dilated with eye drops to inspect the eye behind the iris. During a dilated exam, the eye doctor examines the lens, vitreous, retina, and optic nerve head, often using special lenses. It is during this dilated exam that cataracts, glaucoma, diabetic retinopathy, and age-related macular degeneration can be detected, along with more uncommon eye problems such as tumors, retinal detachments, and vascular abnormalities.

If problems are noted in this comprehensive exam, then other tests may be ordered by the eye doctor. For example, computerized visual field testing is commonly done for glaucoma and other causes of vision loss. Computed tomography (CT scans) and magnetic resonance imaging (MRI scans) of the orbits and brain are performed if problems are suspected in the visual pathways behind the eye that cannot be seen in an eye exam. Photographs of the eyes may be taken, and dye tests to determine blood flow inside the eyes may also be performed.

http://www.aao.org **http:**//www.opted.org **http:**//www.aoa.org
http://www.oaa.org **http:**//www.ama-assn.org

3 · Common Vision Problems

Nearsightedness

JENNIFER S. WEIZER, M.D.

What Is It? · Nearsightedness, or myopia, is the ability to see clearly up close but not at a distance without glasses or contact lenses. The cause of nearsightedness is unknown but it tends to run in families. It is the most common vision problem in the United States, affecting more than 25% of the population.

Nearsightedness usually begins in childhood or early adolescence and progresses until the late teens or early twenties, when it stabilizes. Acquired nearsightedness is much less common and can be caused by many eye diseases which are discussed elsewhere in this book.

Anatomically there are two types of nearsightedness. In axial myopia the eyeball is elongated rather than spherical. Therefore, light rays entering the eye focus in front of the retina instead of right on it. In refractive myopia the refractive power of the cornea or lens is too strong, causing the same effect.

Occasionally a person may be so nearsighted that he or she is at risk for developing other eye diseases. This condition is called high myopia and is defined as a refractive error of more than −6.00 to −8.00 diopters. A high myope may have a higher risk of retinal detachment, choroidal neovascularization, or glaucoma.

Symptoms: What You May Experience · Your vision is always blurred at distance but clear when looking at things up close. A nearsighted child who is not wearing glasses or contact lenses may sit too close to the blackboard or television, squint frequently, or be unaware of distant objects.

Examination Findings: What the Doctor Looks For · You will be unable to read the eye chart at a distance during the exam. If tests

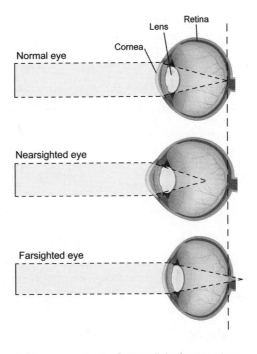

5 Top: normal eye. Center: light focuses too far forward in nearsighted eye. Right: light focuses too far back in farsighted eye.

indicate that glasses are likely to correct the problem, your eye doctor may then write a prescription for glasses or contact lenses.

What You Can Do · There is no proven way to prevent nearsightedness. You should simply be aware of its symptoms so that if nearsightedness develops, you can be examined by an eye doctor.

When to Call the Doctor · Nearsightedness usually develops in children, so parents, teachers, and health care workers should be alert to the symptoms. A child who has difficulty seeing distant objects should see an eye doctor promptly to prevent the development of a lazy eye (amblyopia) and to exclude other causes of blurred vision.

Treatment · Properly prescribed glasses and contact lenses can correct nearsightedness. Some people may benefit from refractive surgery. Annual eye exams are recommended, especially for those with high myopia, because nearsighted people can develop retinal tears and detachments which they may not notice.

Prognosis: Will I See Better? · Most nearsightedness can be fully corrected with glasses or contact lenses.

http://www.nlm.nih.gov/medlineplus/ency/article/001023.htm
http://www.eyemdlink.com/Condition.asp?ConditionID=293

Farsightedness

INDER PAUL SINGH, M.D. · PRATAP CHALLA, M.D.

What Is It? · Farsightedness, or hyperopia, is a condition in which distant objects are usually seen clearly but close objects are blurred. Just as a camera uses lenses to properly focus light on film, the human eye uses the cornea and the lens to focus images on the retina. In farsightedness, the image that falls on the retina is blurred because the light entering the eye is focused behind the retina instead of directly on it. This condition is caused by a cornea that is flatter than normal, a lens in the eye that is not strong enough, or an eyeball that is shorter than average. Approximately 25% of the general population is farsighted.

Many infants are born farsighted but lose their farsightedness by the teenage years. Children and young adults with mild or moderate hyperopia are often able to see clearly because their natural lens can change its shape, or accommodate, to focus on near objects. As farsighted people get older, however, their ability to accommodate declines as the lens becomes less flexible. Eventually, glasses or contact lenses may be required to correct their farsightedness.

Symptoms: What You May Experience · In adults, the vision is blurred at near but may be clearer at distance. You may notice eyestrain or fatigue, especially when reading. A farsighted child who is not wearing glasses or contact lenses may not notice any difficulty seeing up close because of accommodation, but in some farsighted children, eye crossing (strabismus) may occur.

Examination Findings: What the Doctor Looks For · The eye doctor will test your vision and your need for glasses (refraction). In children, the pupils may be dilated to relax accommodation before refraction is performed. Farsightedness is rarely diagnosed in school vision screenings, which typically only test the ability to see distant objects.

What You Can Do · There is no proven way to prevent farsightedness from developing. You should be aware of its symptoms so if farsightedness develops, you can be examined by an eye doctor.

When to Call the Doctor · If you notice blurry vision close up but not at a distance, eye strain, or eye fatigue, you should call your eye doctor. Children should have an eye exam at least once by the age of six to diagnose any farsightedness or other eye problems.

Treatment · Treating farsightedness depends on several factors, including your age and daily activities. Young patients may or may not require glasses or contact lenses, depending on their ability to compensate for their farsightedness with accommodation. Older patients often benefit from glasses or contact lenses, which may only be necessary for reading if their farsightedness is mild. Some farsighted adults may benefit from refractive surgery as another treatment option.

Prognosis: Will I See Better? · Most farsightedness can be fully corrected with glasses or contact lenses.

http://www.eyemdlink.com/Condition.asp?ConditionID=229
http://www.nlm.nih.gov/medlineplus/ency/article/001020.htm

Astigmatism

PRIYATHAM S. METTU, M.D.

What Is It? · Astigmatism is an irregular curvature of the corneal surface of the eye. Instead of being round or spherical, like a basketball, the corneal surface is longer in certain axes, like a football. In eyes with astigmatism, light rays are not bent normally as they enter the eye, preventing the formation of one image at a single point. Most people have some degree of astigmatism, but severe cases can be associated with diseases such as keratoconus or corneal scarring.

Symptoms: What You May Experience · You might notice that your vision is blurred when looking at objects either near or far without glasses or contact lenses. In some cases, astigmatism can be associated with headaches or eyestrain.

Examination Findings: What the Doctor Looks For · Your doctor looks for blurry vision that is improved by looking through lenses of various powers when the doctor tests for glasses as part of the standard eye exam.

What You Can Do · There is no way to prevent astigmatism from occurring.

When to Call the Doctor · People with blurry or distorted vision should be seen promptly by an eye doctor to identify the condition and exclude nearsightedness or farsightedness, which can occur in combination with astigmatism.

Treatment · Astigmatism can usually be corrected with eyeglasses or contact lenses, including soft toric, gas-permeable, or hard contact lenses. In some cases astigmatism can also be corrected by refractive surgery. Astigmatism caused by advanced keratoconus may require a corneal transplant.

Prognosis: Will I See Better? · Most astigmatism can be fully corrected with the above treatments.

http://www.allaboutvision.com/conditions/astigmatism.htm
http://www.nlm.nih.gov/medlineplus/ency/article/001015.htm

Presbyopia

PRIYATHAM S. METTU, M.D.

What Is It? · Presbyopia is a decrease in the ability to see near objects. It is an expected part of the aging process. Normally, muscle

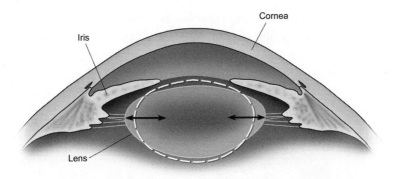

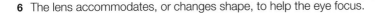

6 The lens accommodates, or changes shape, to help the eye focus.

fibers attached to the lens contract to change the shape of the lens, allowing near objects to come into focus. This is called accommodation. With increasing age, the lens hardens and loses elasticity, becoming less able to change its shape as each eye accommodates for near vision.

Symptoms: What You May Experience · As you reach middle age (the mid-40s), you will likely start to experience blurry vision when attempting to read, and you may find that you have to hold reading materials farther away to see them clearly. Additional symptoms may include eyestrain or headache.

Examination Findings: What the Doctor Looks For · Presbyopia is readily detected as part of a standard eye exam. Your doctor may test the ability of each eye to accommodate to near vision by bringing an object closer and closer to the eye until the vision blurs.

What You Can Do · Presbyopia affects nearly all adults to some degree as they age. It is not preventable.

When to Call the Doctor · Presbyopia typically becomes most apparent during the mid-40s. It may occur at a slightly younger age for farsighted people or at an older age for the nearsighted. You should see an eye doctor when you notice that you are no longer able to read or perform near tasks comfortably.

Treatment · Presbyopia can typically be corrected with eyeglasses, which include reading glasses, bifocals, and progressive addition lenses, or with multifocal contact lenses. Over-the-counter reading glasses are an option for those whose distance vision does not require glasses. In select cases, refractive surgery can aid in the correction of presbyopia.

Prognosis: Will I See Better? · Eyeglasses and contact lenses can usually fully correct presbyopia. However, you may need a more powerful reading prescription as you grow older, since changes in the lens and attached muscle fibers continue.

http://www.aoa.org/conditions/presbyopia.asp
http://www.allaboutvision.com/conditions/presbyopia.htm

Colorblindness

INDER PAUL SINGH, M.D. · PRATAP CHALLA, M.D.

What Is It? · Colorblindness is a deficiency in the way colors are seen. With this vision problem, a person has difficulty distinguishing certain colors, such as red and green or blue and yellow. Red-green color deficiency is by far the most common form of colorblindness; a less common form is blue-yellow color deficiency. It is extremely rare to not be able to distinguish any color at all — this disease is called achromatopsia and usually accompanies other serious eye problems.

The cone cells of the retina are responsible for allowing us to see color. Each cone contains a specific pigment — either red, green, or blue. Colorblindness occurs when one of these color pigments is missing or defective. The deficiency may be partial (affecting only some shades of a color) or complete (affecting all shades of the color).

Usually people with color vision problems are born with them. Colorblindness affects more men than women, because it is usually caused by an X-linked gene. If this type of gene is passed from a mother to her children, only her sons have a 50% chance of having disease effects, while her daughters will tend to be unaffected carriers. A colorblind father passes the disease gene only to his daughters, who are again unaffected carriers. Approximately one in twelve men has at least some color perception problems.

Colorblindness sometimes occurs after a person is born. Some other diseases that can lead to colorblindness include retinitis pigmentosa, optic neuropathy, Alzheimer's disease, diabetes mellitus, glaucoma, leukemia, liver disease, chronic alcoholism, age-related macular degeneration, multiple sclerosis, Parkinson's disease, and sickle-cell anemia. Injuries or strokes that damage the retina, optic nerve, or particular areas of the brain can also lead to colorblindness. Some medications, such as certain antibiotics, barbiturates, anti-tuberculosis drugs, high-blood-pressure medications, and several medications used to treat autoimmune and psychiatric problems, can cause color vision changes as well.

Symptoms: What You May Experience · Certain colors may appear gray, or two colors that appear different to normal people may appear similar to a person with colorblindness. People who are born with color vision problems may not notice the difficulty that they have in distinguishing certain colors when they are young.

Examination Findings: What the Doctor Looks For · The eye doctor will perform a color vision test, of which several types are available. Some color tests ask you to distinguish a colored figure or number from a background, while other tests involve identifying and grouping similar colors together. All color tests are designed to identify the type of colorblindness, if it is present.

What You Can Do · There is no known prevention for colorblindness. Because the disease is often inherited, tell your eye doctor if it is present in your family.

When to Call the Doctor · If you notice difficulty telling colors apart, call your eye doctor. A new color vision problem that was not present at birth may be a sign of another disease or a problem with medication. Also, parents should be alert to symptoms of colorblindness in their children.

Treatment · Unfortunately, most inherited colorblindness cannot be cured. Most people with color vision problems compensate well for their deficiency and rely on color cues and details that are not consciously evident to those with normal color vision, sometimes with the help of adaptive equipment. Wearing glasses with tinted lenses can sometimes help those with achromatopsia who are sensitive to bright light.

Noninherited color blindness that has a specific cause is treated by treating the underlying problem.

Prognosis: Will I See Better? · Inherited colorblindness usually does not change over the course of a person's lifetime. The prognosis for colorblindness that occurs after birth depends on the underlying problem. For instance, if the colorblindness is due to a medication, stopping the medication under a physician's guidance can often make color vision return to normal.

http://www.preventblindness.org/eye_problems/colorvision.html
http://www.eyemdlink.com/Condition.asp?ConditionID=116

4 · Options for Correcting Vision

Glasses

HELEN CHANDLER, O.D.

People are often surprised to learn how many options they have when filling their eyeglass prescriptions. Among these options are various lens designs. The basic design is called "single vision," an all-purpose lens designed to correct distance vision. Multifocal lenses are designed to correct both distance vision and near vision; the upper portion of the lens is focused for distance vision, while the shorter focal point of the bottom portion is used for near tasks such as reading. Multifocal lenses can be bifocals, trifocals, or progressive lenses. Bifocals have one line separating the top part of the lens, for distance, from the bottom portion, for close viewing. Trifocal lenses focus light in three areas: distance vision, intermediate vision, and near vision. One disadvantage of bifocals and trifocals is the abrupt demarcation between each area of the lens. Progressive lenses alleviate this problem by replacing the sharp divisions with a smooth transition between distance and near vision. By eliminating the lines between the focal areas, progressive lenses are also cosmetically desirable; however, each focal area is relatively small because more lens space is used for the transitional areas.

Lens material is another option. Traditionally eyeglass lenses were made of glass. Today, however, most lenses are plastic. Plastic eyeglasses are lighter, more flexible, and less likely to shatter. One type of plastic lens is a "high-index" lens, which is especially thin and light. High-index lenses are most often recommended when the need for visual correction is high, because they reduce the dreaded "coke-bottle" appearance of thick glasses. Eye care professionals recommend another option, polycarbonate lenses, for patients who wear glasses for sports or other potentially hazard-

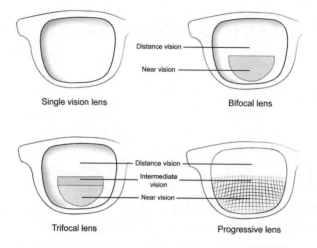

7 Top left: single-vision glasses lens. Top right: bifocal glasses lens. Bottom left: trifocal glasses lens. Bottom right: progressive glasses lens.

ous activities. Polycarbonate is a safety lens material that is highly impact resistant.

Protective coatings for lenses are another option. Anti-reflective coatings reduce unwanted reflections and help to alleviate glare or eyestrain, especially during night driving. Another type of coating helps to protect the eyes from ultraviolet (uv) light. With the exception of polycarbonate lenses, most lenses are not inherently uv protective. This extra coating eliminates uv light, protecting the eyes from harmful radiation.

One simple option for lenses that correct vision while protecting the eyes from sunlight is prescription sunglasses. For patients who would rather wear only one set of eyeglasses indoors and out, photochromatic lenses are a good option. Photochromatic lenses change tint according to the amount of light they receive, darkening in the sunlight and lightening indoors.

http://www.eyemdlink.com/Test.asp?TestID=18
http://www.visionchannel.net/refractivecorrection/

Contact Lenses

HELEN CHANDLER, O.D.

Contact lenses correct nearsightedness, farsightedness, and astigmatism. Some contacts may even aid in the correction of presbyopia. The benefits of wearing contacts instead of glasses include cosmetic considerations, better peripheral or side vision (and in some cases better vision overall), and visual correction during sports.

A contact lens prescription requires more detail than a prescription for eyeglasses. In addition to the information in an eyeglass prescription, a contact lens prescription also includes the fitting parameters, such as the size and curvature of the contact lens, which directly affect the health of the cornea and conjunctiva. Contact lenses are medical devices regulated by the Food and Drug Administration (FDA) and are prescribed by eye doctors only after the health of the eye has been assessed.

Not everyone can wear contact lenses. People who have severe dry eyes, severe eye allergies, active eye infection, or a compromised immune system, among other conditions, cannot safely wear contact lenses.

Because contact lenses are in direct contact with the eye, they pose an inherent risk of infection or injury to the eye. Contact lenses must be cared for properly and worn according to the eye doctor's recommendations. If these recommendations are followed, then contacts are generally safe. If patients misuse their contacts, they can develop corneal abrasions, infectious keratitis, conjunctivitis (pink eye), or other eye problems. In severe cases of infection, permanent corneal scarring may occur. For these reasons, it is important for all contact lens wearers to be examined by an eye doctor at least annually.

Contact lenses may be classified in several ways. Soft lenses are made of flexible plastic, while gas-permeable, or "hard," lenses are composed of rigid plastic. The advantages of soft lenses are their disposability and comfort. The advantages of gas-permeable lenses include better vision for some patients who have astigmatism or irregular corneas, greater availability of oxygen, better tear flow to the cornea, and durability. Gas-permeable lenses are generally not as comfortable initially to patients. Soft lenses require solutions for cleaning, disinfecting, and storage different from those used for gas-permeable lenses. Contrary to popular belief, many patients who have astigmatism can wear soft contacts, because toric lenses (soft lenses that correct astigmatism) have been developed extensively in recent years. However, patients who have keratoconus, high astigmatism, or irregular astigmatism often benefit from gas-permeable lenses.

Contact lenses can also be classified according to their replacement schedule. "Conventional" lenses are designed to be replaced yearly. "Disposable" lenses are designed to be replaced more frequently, such as quarterly, monthly, biweekly, weekly, or daily. It is generally healthier for the eye to replace lenses frequently. Disposable lenses may also be better for patients with mild eye allergies.

Contact lenses can also be classified by the length of time they can be safely worn each day. "Daily wear" lenses are worn only during waking hours. "Extended wear" lenses are approved by the FDA for wear during sleep. Although sleeping with lenses on may be convenient, it is generally not advisable. If you sleep with lenses on, the risk of infection is much higher, and long-term corneal health may be compromised.

Contact lenses should always be handled with proper care. You should always wash your hands before handling your lenses. Because of the great variety in eye-care products, only solutions recommended by your eye-care professional should be used. Contacts should never be exposed to saliva or tap water. Eye cosmetics should be applied only after insertion of the lens. If the eye becomes red, swollen, or otherwise causes discomfort, patients should remove the lens immediately and report the problem to their eye doctor.

http://www.fda.gov/cdrh/consumer/buycontactqa.html
http://www.aao.org/aao/advocacy/federal/regulatory/
  deregulation_statement.cfm

Refractive Surgery

ALAN N. CARLSON, M.D.

What Is Refractive Surgery? · Refractive surgery, or vision correction surgery, is a family of surgical techniques designed to improve a person's unaided vision (vision without glasses or contact lenses). LASIK (laser-assisted in situ keratomileusis) is the most commonly performed refractive surgery procedure: its rapid growth has made it one of the most common surgeries in the United States. Each year two million LASIK procedures are performed worldwide.

The goal of improving one's vision without the need for glasses or contact lenses is certainly not new. The intraocular lens implant, which is inserted during cataract surgery, was designed with this goal in mind over half a century ago. Radial keratotomy (RK) is an early refractive surgery technique designed to change the focusing power of the eye by making precise cuts in the cornea (the clear, front part of the eyeball). While RK is successful in correcting nearsightedness, our surgical options have progressed greatly in recent years, thanks to an array of technological advancements. Among these are sophisticated procedures in which skilled ophthalmologists use an extremely precise laser to treat nearsightedness, farsightedness, and astigmatism by reshaping the surface of the eye.

Who Might Consider Refractive Surgery? · The ideal person to consider refractive surgery is someone who feels that his or her quality of life would be much better with less dependence on glasses or contact lenses. People whose work environment is hazardous for wearing glasses or contact lenses, such as law enforcement officers, firefighters, some athletes, or those working around toxic chemicals or in dusty or dirty environments, might also consider refractive surgery. Patients completely satisfied with their glasses or contact lenses are not considered good candidates for vision correction surgery.

If you are considering refractive surgery, your glasses or contact lens prescription must be stable, without changing significantly during the previous year. While most significant changes in refraction occur before the age of 15, some patients with extreme nearsightedness may continue to experience changes until they stabilize at an older age. The Food and Drug Administration has approved LASIK for patients over the age of 21; under special circumstances, surgery can sometimes be performed at younger ages. There is no upper age limit for surgery as long as you do not have a disease that might affect your outcome or recovery from vision correction surgery.

Patients who should not have vision correction surgery include those with a history of herpes virus eye infection (herpes simplex or zoster), or systemic illnesses such as rheumatoid arthritis or systemic lupus erythematosus, that may adversely affect healing of the eye. Refractive surgeons also examine candidates to exclude those who might end up with a cornea that is too thin, too flat, or too steep after surgery, which can affect the quality of vision. Before surgery, soft contact lens wearers are advised to avoid wearing their lenses for two weeks. Toric soft contact lenses and rigid, gas-permeable contact lenses must be discontinued for even longer, depending on how long they have been worn.

It is important to remember that refractive surgery is not for everyone. Some people will need to wait for improvements in technology before they can be considered appropriate candidates for surgery. Even if you are technically an ideal candidate for refractive surgery, you should thoroughly understand the surgical procedure, postoperative limitations, and potential risks associated with the surgery, while maintaining reasonable expectations of the results.

How Does Refractive Surgery Work? · The most common types of refractive surgery change the focusing properties of the eye by reshaping the cornea with a laser. The new shape of the cornea is designed to simulate the focusing power of a properly fit contact lens. The first step in refractive surgery techniques is taking many precise measurements of the eye and then using a computer to calculate the precise amount of corneal reshaping to be done by the laser.

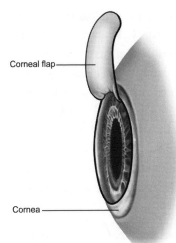

Corneal flap

Cornea

8 A flap is made in the cornea during LASIK surgery.

The high degree of precision needed for this type of surgery requires a specialized excimer laser capable of removing amounts of tissue that measure only 1/100,000 of an inch. Reshaping the cornea can occur on the corneal surface—as in photorefractive keratectomy (PRK) or laser epithelial keratomileusis (LASEK)—or under a protective, surgically created corneal flap (as in LASIK).

The most exciting recent advance in refractive surgery individualizes each patient's treatment by using wavefront technology to remove high-order aberrations. These aberrations are tiny optical imperfections that can distort vision and are not correctable by glasses or contact lenses. The customized approach to laser vision correction has also been shown to reduce vision problems associated with glare and night driving. Wavefront refractive surgery requires a specialized series of eye measurements and consultation with your refractive surgeon to see if you qualify.

What Are the Risks of Refractive Surgery? · The Food and Drug Administration states that laser vision correction surgery is a safe and effective procedure for appropriate candidates who fit specific treatment guidelines. No surgical procedure is risk-free, however. There is a 1–2% chance of having a "minor" complication that may slow your recovery, lead to small disturbances in vision, possibly delay surgery, or require additional surgery. There is a 0.2–0.4% chance of having a "major" complication that may permanently reduce your correctable vision. A thorough consultation with a surgeon before surgery helps to exclude those patients considered at high risk for complications.

While vision correction surgery is not believed to lead to or worsen cataracts, glaucoma, or age-related macular degeneration, it also does not prevent these conditions. Patients are reminded to continue routine follow-up eye examinations after refractive surgery.

How Long Do the Results of Refractive Surgery Last? · Currently available laser techniques yield more stable results than some older surgical techniques such as radial keratotomy. Overall, 6–8% of patients undergoing laser vision correction surgery will need some additional correction, referred to as an "enhancement" procedure. The likelihood of needing an enhancement procedure increases for patients who initially require large amounts of correction.

What Other Factors Are Important When Considering Refractive Surgery? · It is essential to do your research and seek a thorough evaluation from a qualified and experienced facility. When you are faced with aggressive marketing campaigns and attempts to lure potential patients with discount pricing, it is important to remember that you are contemplating eye surgery. Facilities offering the latest technology, a top-notch staff, and surgeons of the highest caliber will tend to stay in business over time and will not compensate for their shortcomings with aggressive marketing and deeply discounted pricing. Finding a surgeon and a facility with which you feel comfortable is a major part of having successful refractive surgery.

http://www.aao.org/ **http://**www.ascrs.org
http://www.fda.gov/cdrh/lasik/

Protective Eyewear

HELEN CHANDLER, O.D.

The National Society for the Prevention of Blindness has estimated that 90% of eye injuries are preventable. Eye injuries may result in short-term visual disability or may be permanently disabling, yet most injuries are entirely preventable with proper eyewear.

Eye injuries may occur in many ways. Direct impact from an object, heat, chemicals, dust, and radiation represent the most common hazards. Each hazard can be significantly reduced by specific protective eyewear.

Non-safety eyeglasses with either glass or plastic lenses can be hazardous because breakage can cause direct eye injury. Most lens breakage occurs from either the crushing impact of large, slow-moving objects or the shattering impact of small, high-speed objects. Polycarbonate is the only appropriate lens material for safety eyewear.

The American National Standards Institute (ANSI) is the source of guidance for selecting eyewear for specific hazards. ANSI also establishes the criteria for the production of lenses by optical laboratories. These standards themselves are not laws, but they are adopted by governmental agencies such as the Occupational Safety and Health Administration and the Food and Drug Administration. ANSI has created different standards for "dress eyewear" and "industrial eyewear." These standards include specified impact resistance and a minimum thickness of lenses. Frames must also meet standards of impact resistance, non-inflammability, and corrosion resistance. For industrial safety eyewear, frames must be labeled "Z87" to indicate that they meet ANSI standards.

For more information on protective eyewear appropriate for your activities, consult your eye-care professional.

http://www.medem.com/medlb/article_detaillb.cfm?article_ID=
ZZZEGMLPSKC&sub_cat=32

http://www.preventblindness.org/safety/recommended.html

Blepharitis

JENNIFER S. WEIZER, M.D. · JOHN J. MICHON, M.D.

What Is It? · Blepharitis means inflammation of the eyelid margins, or edges where the eyelashes grow. This condition is one of the most common causes of eye irritation. Blepharitis can result from bacterial infection, abnormal oil gland secretions, or a combination of both. In bacterial blepharitis, certain bacteria live in the eyelids and cause irritation. Abnormal oil gland secretions result when the eyelid glands that make oil for the normal tear film produce too much oil that is overly thick, also causing eye irritation. Blepharitis is often found in patients with dry eye syndrome and rosacea. Moderate to severe blepharitis can cause irritation of the conjunctiva and the cornea, as the eyelids rub against the surface of the eyeball.

Symptoms: What You May Experience · You may notice eye burning, itching, mild redness, the feeling that something is in the eye, or crusting around the eyelashes that is particularly worse upon awakening.

Examination Findings: What the Doctor Looks for · Your eye doctor will examine your eyes with a slit lamp to look for crusting and debris around the base of your eyelashes, as well as clogging of your eyelid oil glands. He or she will look for signs of corneal or conjunctival irritation, as well as signs of dry eye.

What You Can Do · If you notice mild symptoms of eye irritation, you can try the following lid hygiene techniques:

1. Moisten a clean washcloth with warm water, wring out the excess, and use the washcloth as a warm compress for your eyelids while keeping your eyes closed. This should be done twice daily for at least five minutes at a time.

2. After using the warm compress, place a drop of tear-free baby shampoo on the damp washcloth and use it to gently massage the base of your eyelashes while your eyes are closed. Rinse afterward.

Also, preservative-free artificial tear drops, which are available over the counter, can be used as frequently as necessary.

When to Call the Doctor · If your symptoms of eye irritation are not improved with lid hygiene or artificial tears, or if your symptoms are severe, call your eye doctor. If you notice decreased vision or eye discharge, call your eye doctor promptly, since these symptoms may signify a more serious eye problem.

Treatment · Besides recommending lid hygiene and preservative-free artificial tears, your eye doctor may prescribe antibiotic ointment to be applied to the edges of your eyelids if your blepharitis is moderate to severe. In some cases that do not improve, he or she may prescribe an antibiotic, such as doxycycline, to be taken by mouth for several weeks. Rarely, steroid eye drops may be necessary for a short course.

Prognosis: Will I See Better? · Blepharitis is a chronic condition that can be controlled but is usually not completely cured. Lid hygiene techniques may need to be performed consistently for days to weeks before you notice less eye irritation, and antibiotic courses may also need to be repeated over time. With faithful use of these treatments, however, most patients will notice an improvement in their symptoms.

http://www.nei.nih.gov/health/blepharitis/
http://www.eyemdlink.com/Condition.asp?ConditionID=76

Ocular Rosacea

JENNIFER S. WEIZER, M.D. · JOHN J. MICHON, M.D.

What Is It? · Rosacea is an inflammatory disease of the oil glands on the face, neck, and shoulders. In ocular rosacea, the oil glands in the eyelid margins are particularly affected. Rosacea affects mostly people aged 30–50, and women are slightly more prone to the disease than men.

The inflamed eyelid oil glands that are affected in ocular rosacea can cause severe blepharitis, frequent formation of styes, and irritation of the eye's surface which is often more severe than in cases of blepharitis where rosacea is not the cause. This surface irritation can result in conjunctivitis, corneal ulcers, episcleritis, or even uveitis. Over time, abnormal new blood vessels can grow onto the normally clear cornea, and corneal scarring can result.

Symptoms: What You May Experience · You may notice burning, itching, or redness in your eyes, the feeling that something is in your eye, frequent styes, and blurred vision. These blepharitis-like symptoms are usually accompanied by spidery facial blood vessels, facial redness, and adult acne in rosacea. Light-complexioned persons with rosacea may notice facial flushing, especially when drinking alcohol or hot beverages. Rosacea that is long-standing can result in thickened skin and enlargement of the nose.

Examination Findings: What the Doctor Looks For · Your eye doctor will examine your face for the abnormal blood vessels, flushed complexion, and adult acne associated with rosacea. He or she will examine your eyes with a slit lamp to look for signs of severe blepharitis as well as any irritation or inflammation of the front surface of your eye.

What You Can Do · There is no proven way to prevent the occurrence of rosacea. Lid hygiene techniques and preservative-free artificial tears that are useful for regular blepharitis may help the symptoms of rosacea somewhat, but usually cannot treat rosacea completely.

When to Call the Doctor · If you notice eye irritation that is not relieved by artificial tears and lid hygiene, especially when accompanied by abnormal facial flushing or adult acne, you should see your eye doctor. If you also notice decreased vision or eye discharge, make sure to see your eye doctor promptly: these symptoms may signify a severe eye problem.

Treatment · The mainstay of rosacea treatment is antibiotics such as doxycycline taken by mouth, which may need to be continued for years at a low dose. Although rosacea is not caused by a bacterial infection, doxycycline and other related antibiotics also help to control inflammation of the oil glands. In certain cases another antibiotic, called metronidazole and available in gel form, can help treat the facial redness. Rosacea-induced keratitis, corneal ulcers (as long as they are not caused by an infection), and abnormal blood vessels in the cornea may be treated with a course of steroid eye drops. In cases of severe corneal scarring from rosacea, a corneal transplant may be considered with caution if the overall level of inflammation is controlled.

Prognosis: Will I See Better? · Rosacea is difficult to cure completely. The treatments are intended to control the inflammation of the oil glands as much as possible, and most people with rosacea who are treated with antibiotics notice at least some improvement in inflammation and irritation of the eyes and face. Rosacea patients who require a corneal transplant because of severe disease are often prone to transplant failure over time, because the underlying inflammation from the rosacea can cause the body to reject the transplanted cornea.

www.rosacea.org **http://**www.nlm.nih.gov/medlineplus/rosacea.html

Stye and Chalazion

JENNIFER S. WEIZER, M.D. · JOHN J. MICHON, M.D.

What Is It? · A stye, or hordeolum, is a nodule of inflammation that forms a bump in the eyelid and is associated with a bacterial infection. A stye usually begins to form when an oil gland in the eyelid margin becomes clogged. A pocket of bacterial infection, or an abscess, then develops in the clogged oil gland. Very rarely, the infection can spread from the eyelid to other parts of the face. Persons with blepharitis are especially prone to developing styes.

In contrast to a stye, a chalazion is a nodule of inflammation that forms a bump in the eyelid without associated infection. Chalazia tend to be present longer than styes, and they are usually less tender and red. Some styes develop into chalazia after the body clears the infection but not the inflammation.

Symptoms: What You May Experience · With a stye, you will notice a bump in your eyelid that develops over several days. The bump is usually tender and red. With a chalazion, the bump that forms in your eyelid will often take longer to form. It is usually only slightly tender to the touch and is less red than a stye. Your vision may be slightly blurred if the chalazion presses on your eyeball, causing astigmatism (an irregular curvature of the cornea).

Examination Findings: What the Doctor Looks for · Your eye doctor will examine your eyelids to determine if a stye or chalazion is present. He or she may flip your upper eyelids inside out to see if the stye or chalazion is on the inside surface of the eyelid. He or she may also examine your eyelid margins with a slit lamp to see if blepharitis, which may have caused the stye or chalazion to form, is present.

What You Can Do · If you have blepharitis, perform regular lid hygiene with warm compresses and lid scrubs to control the blepharitis and reduce your chance of developing a stye or chalazion. If a stye or chalazion does form, using warm compresses several times a day may help it to heal faster. To make a warm compress, wet a washcloth with warm water, wring out the excess, and place the cloth over your closed eyelids for at least five minutes.

When to Call the Doctor · If you have a stye or chalazion that does not improve after several days of warm compresses or becomes very large and bothersome, call your ophthalmologist. If the redness and swelling spread beyond the eyelid or if you develop a fever, call your ophthalmologist immediately. If you have chalazia that keep reoccurring, see your eye doctor, because some rare serious eye diseases can present in this way.

Treatment · If a stye is very large or does not improve with frequent warm compresses, your ophthalmologist may cut it open to let the contents drain out. Chalazia that have been present for several weeks or months are slower to improve on their own and can

also benefit from surgical drainage. Antibiotics alone are generally not helpful for styes or chalazia, unless the infection spreads
to other parts of the face.

Drainage of a stye or chalazion is done in the office after local
numbing medicine is injected into the eyelid. In many cases, the
stye or chalazion can be cut open from the inside of the eyelid so
the wound is not visible, rather than through the eyelid skin. Over
the next several days, your ophthalmologist may prescribe an antibiotic eye ointment while the stye or chalazion continues to heal.

Prognosis: Will I See Better? · Most styes heal over several days
on their own without requiring surgical drainage, and frequent
warm compresses can speed this healing. Some chalazia also heal
on their own, but others are slower to improve without being cut
open and drained. Whether the stye or chalazion heals on its own
or with surgical drainage, the eyelid generally heals well afterward
with little or no scarring.

http://www.med.umich.edu/1libr/pa/pa_stye_hhg.htm
http://www.nlm.nih.gov/medlineplus/ency/article/001006.htm

Dacryocystitis: Tear Duct and Sac Infection

JENNIFER S. WEIZER, M.D. · JOHN J. MICHON, M.D.
What Is It? · Dacryocystitis is an infection of the tear drainage system. Tears are normally made by the lacrimal gland under the
upper eyelid and drain out through a system of ducts to the lacrimal sac and out into the nose. If there is a blockage in this drainage
system, tears cannot drain out properly, allowing bacteria to grow
in the ducts or lacrimal sac and cause dacryocystitis. Such blockages of the tear drainage system may be due to aging, injury, sinus
disease, inflammatory diseases, or scarring from previous episodes
of dacryocystitis. In severe cases, the infection can spread to the
surrounding skin and other areas of the face or orbit.

Symptoms: What You May Experience · If you have a blockage of
your tear drainage system, you may notice excessive watering of
your eyes. If infection develops, resulting in dacryocystitis, you

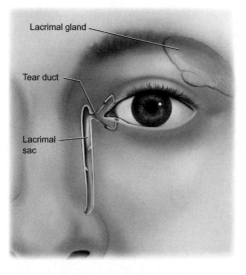

Lacrimal gland

Tear duct

Lacrimal sac

9 Tears flow from the lacrimal gland, lubricate the surface of the eyeball, and drain through the tear ducts and lacrimal sac into the nose.

may notice redness, pain, and swelling of the skin below the inner corner of the eye, toward the nose. The eye itself may also feel irritated.

Examination Findings: What the Doctor Looks for · The eye doctor will examine the area where the tear drainage system is located, just below the inner corner of the eye. He or she will look for redness and swelling of the skin, as well as touch the area to check for tenderness and to see if pus comes out of the tear duct.

What You Can Do · If you notice pain, redness, and swelling of the area of skin just below the inner corner of the eye, apply warm compresses frequently and call your eye doctor promptly.

When to Call the Doctor · If you develop constant, excessive tearing, see your ophthalmologist, because blockage of the tear duct system can be treated before infection develops. Once you notice pain, redness, and swelling of the skin below the inner corner of the eye, see your eye doctor promptly so treatment can be started before the infection spreads.

Treatment · Active dacryocystitis is treated with antibiotics taken by mouth. Warm compresses can help the infection resolve faster.

If the infection has already spread to the orbit or other areas of the face, intravenous antibiotics and hospitalization may be needed. If an abscess, or pus pocket, forms in the tear drainage system, your ophthalmologist may need to cut it open so that the infection can drain out.

Once the active infection is controlled, your ophthalmologist may flush salt solution though your tear drainage system to see if a blockage is present. If the salt solution does not flush through because of a blockage, surgery may be needed to create a drain for the tears so that dacryocystitis does not reoccur. This operation is called dacryocystorhinostomy (DCR) and is performed in the operating room under sedation or general anesthesia. In a DCR, a direct passage for tears is created between the lacrimal sac and the inside of the nose.

Prognosis: Will I See Better? · Most cases of dacryocystitis resolve well with antibiotic treatment. Because the infection is caused by a blocked tear drainage system in most cases, dacryocystitis often reoccurs if the blockage is not treated. A DCR will fix the blockage in over 90% of patients.

http://www.eyemdlink.com/Condition.asp?ConditionID=18
http://www.emedicine.com/OPH/topic708.htm

Drooping Eyelids

JENNIFER S. WEIZER, M.D. · JOHN J. MICHON, M.D.

What Is It? · Drooping upper eyelids, known as ptosis, can occur at birth, or more commonly in adulthood. Newborns with ptosis usually have underdevelopment of the muscle that lifts the upper eyelid, while adult ptosis has a variety of causes. The most common cause is age-induced stretching of the muscle that lifts the upper eyelid, but injury, muscle diseases, or nerve diseases of the muscle or upper eyelid are also potential causes of ptosis.

Besides being a cosmetic problem, drooping upper eyelids can block upward vision and, if the eyelids are low enough, even central vision. In the case of nerve problems that result in drooping upper eyelids, ptosis can be a sign of a more serious neurologic problem. In infants, drooping upper eyelids can cause amblyopia (poor visual development) by blocking central vision or causing astigmatism which distorts the vision.

Symptoms: What You May Experience · If your upper eyelids droop, you may notice that your eyelids block your vision when you look upward or even straight ahead. You may have trouble reading, because your eyelids may droop even more when you are looking down at a book. You may also notice forehead tension headaches if you lift your eyebrows with your forehead muscles to help raise your upper eyelids. If your ptosis has a neurologic cause, one upper eyelid may droop more than the other, the droopiness may fluctuate (often becoming worse later in the day), or you may experience double vision.

Examination Findings: What the Doctor Looks for · Your eye doctor will ask questions about how long your upper eyelids have drooped and if the droopiness fluctuates, as well as if you have any muscle or nerve diseases that could cause the droopiness. He or she will measure your eyelid position and test how far you can raise your upper eyelids and if you can close your eyes completely. Your pupils and eye movements will be examined, since nerve damage that causes drooping eyelids can also affect these functions. Your peripheral vision may be checked to determine if your drooping upper eyelids are blocking your upward field of view, and photographs showing your eyelid position may be taken.

What You Can Do · Besides avoiding injury to the upper eyelid and its muscle, there is no way to prevent ptosis from developing.

When to Call the Doctor · If your upper eyelids droop and block your vision, see your ophthalmologist to discuss treatment options. You should see your ophthalmologist especially promptly if the ptosis is present in an infant or child, is new or fluctuates, or is accompanied by unequal pupils or double vision. If the ptosis occurs along with new weakness in other muscles, or difficulty breathing, swallowing, or speaking, go to your local emergency room immediately.

Treatment · The treatment of drooping upper eyelids usually involves surgery in the operating room or minor operating room to repair the droopiness. Your ophthalmologist will choose a surgical technique depending on the amount of ptosis and the function of the muscle that lifts the upper eyelid. Most ptosis repairs are performed with numbing injections and sedation for comfort, although in some cases general anesthesia may be necessary. In some types of ptosis surgery you may be asked to open and close your eyes during the operation, to help the surgeon judge how much to raise your upper eyelids and avoid raising them so much that you cannot close your eyes completely. The ophthalmologist will place stitches to close your eyelid incisions during surgery; these stitches will be removed approximately one week afterward.

Prognosis: Will I See Better? · Most ptosis surgeries are successful. Some patients require more than one surgery to fully correct the ptosis, since it can be difficult to judge the position of the eyelid when the patient is under anesthesia in the operating room.

http://www.nlm.nih.gov/medlineplus/ency/article/001018.htm
http://www.asoprs.org/Pages/ptosis.html

Ectropion and Entropion: Everted and Inverted Eyelids

JENNIFER S. WEIZER, M.D. · JOHN J. MICHON, M.D.

What Is It? · Ectropion means an outward turning of the eyelid margin away from the eyeball. In most cases, the lower eyelid is affected by ectropion. Ectropion usually occurs because the lower eyelid tissues relax with gravity as a person ages; other causes of ectropion include nerve problems, scarring from previous eyelid injury, abnormal growths that pull the eyelid out of position, and developmental defects (in newborns). Besides being a cosmetic issue, ectropion can lead to tearing problems, because the main entrance to the tear drainage system is in the lower eyelid. If this entrance hole no longer sits against the eyeball because the lower eyelid sags outward in ectropion, tears cannot drain properly. Also, these tears may not lubricate the eyeball's surface properly because the droopy lower lid does not hold the tears in place.

Entropion, on the other hand, is an inward turning of the eyelid margin toward the eyeball. As in ectropion, the lower eyelid is most commonly affected. Causes of entropion include aging, eyelid muscle spasms, scarring, and birth defects (in newborns). Most of the problems caused by entropion involve the eyelashes rubbing against the surface of the eyeball as the eyelid turns inward.

Symptoms: What You May Experience · With ectropion, you may see that your lower eyelids sag instead of resting tightly against the eyeball. In entropion, your lower eyelids may curl inward, toward your eyeballs, and your eyelashes may rub against your eyeballs as you blink. Both conditions can cause watering of the eyes, redness, irritation, or burning.

Examination Findings: What the Doctor Looks for · Your eye doctor will examine the position of your eyelids and look for a cause of the ectropion or entropion. He or she will assess the position of your tear drainage system opening in the lower eyelid and check whether your eyelashes are rubbing against your eyeball. With a slit lamp, your eye doctor will examine the surface of your eyeball for tear problems or for damage from inverted eyelashes.

What You Can Do · There is no proven way to avoid developing ectropion or entropion.

When to Call the Doctor · If you notice that your eyelids turn inward or outward, or if you experience excessive watering of the eyes, redness, irritation, or burning, see your eye doctor.

Treatment · Treatment of ectropion and entropion depends on the underlying cause. If age and gravity have caused the lower eyelids to sag outward or turn inward, surgery is often indicated to tighten and restore the eyelids to their natural position. This type of surgery is usually performed in the operating room or minor operating room with sedation and local numbing injections. Some cases of ectropion caused by nerve problems can be treated temporarily if the eyelid nerves are expected to recover. Temporary treatments include lubricating eye drops and ointment, taping of the lower eyelid into position, partial sewing together of the eyelids to help the eyeball stay lubricated, and implantation of a temporary gold weight into the upper eyelid to help the eye close. For entropion, treatments beside eyelid-tightening surgery can include plucking inverted eyelashes and freezing or heating them so that they fall out and do not grow again.

Prognosis: Will I See Better? · Most cases of ectropion and entropion can be improved greatly with treatment. The final outcome depends on the specific cause and extent of eyelid malpositioning.

http://www.asoprs.org/Pages/ectropion.html
http://www.asoprs.org/Pages/entropion.html

Cancers and Benign Lesions of the Eyelids

JENNIFER S. WEIZER, M.D. · JOHN J. MICHON, M.D.

What Is It? · Many growths occur on the eyelids, and these growths can be divided into those that are cancerous (about 15–20% of eyelid growths) and those that are noncancerous, or benign (80–85% of eyelid growths). Most of these growths come from the skin of the eyelid itself. It is important to recognize cancerous eyelid growths so they can be removed, just as skin cancers on other parts of the body should be removed, while benign eyelid growths are generally not harmful.

There are several types of cancer that occur on the eyelids. The most common variety (comprising 90–95% of eyelid cancers) is basal cell carcinoma, which arises from eyelid skin. Squamous cell carcinoma also grows from eyelid skin, while sebaceous cell carcinoma is a rare cancer of the eyelid oil glands. Melanoma is a cancer of the pigmented cells in the skin. In general, the risk that an eyelid lesion is cancerous increases with a history of heavy sun exposure, previous skin cancers, previous radiation, smoking, or a fair complexion.

Benign eyelid lesions, of which there are many types, can be cosmetically unsightly or irritating but pose less risk to the patient's health. Some of these are precancerous, however: over time they can evolve into a cancer.

Symptoms: What You May Experience · You may see a growth on your eyelid. Symptoms suggesting that a growth is cancerous include slow, painless growth, bleeding and crusting of the lesion, color changes, a pearly appearance, changes in the shape of the eyelid margin, loss of eyelashes, and abnormal blood vessels on the lesion.

Examination Findings: What the Doctor Looks for · Your eye doctor will examine your eyelid lesion and decide if there is a risk that it is cancerous.

What You Can Do · Many eyelid growths are not preventable, but you can reduce your risk of developing some (especially many of the cancerous types) by avoiding excessive exposure to the sun and smoking.

When to Call the Doctor · You can see your ophthalmologist for any eyelid lesion that bothers you, but it is especially important to be examined promptly if the lesion is growing, bleeding, crusting, distorting the eyelid, changing color, or causing loss of eyelashes. These signs may suggest that a lesion is cancerous.

Treatment · When your eye doctor examines your eyelid lesion, he or she will decide if cancer is suspected. If the lesion appears small and benign, it can usually be removed in the office. You may require stitches and antibiotic ointment while it heals. If your ophthalmologist suspects an eyelid cancer, he or she will take a sample of the lesion and send it to the laboratory to determine whether cancer is present and, if so, whether the edges of the sample are cancer-free. If the lesion is large or if the edges of the sample still contain cancer, more of the lesion may have to be removed subsequently. Removing large cancers can leave large defects in the eyelid, and in some cases reconstructive surgery performed by a specially trained ophthalmologist or plastic surgeon may be necessary.

Prognosis: Will I See Better? · Many eyelid growths, both cancerous and benign, are easily treated by removing them surgically. Larger or deeper growths may be more difficult to remove because of the defects left where the lesions were. Fortunately, basal cell carcinoma, the most common eyelid cancer, rarely spreads to other areas of the body. Other rarer types of eyelid cancer may behave more aggressively and sometimes require chemotherapy or radiation in addition to surgery.

http://www.asoprs.org/Pages/skincancer.html
http://www.eyemdlink.com/EyeProcedure.asp?EyeProcedureID=38

Blepharospasm

JENNIFER S. WEIZER, M.D. · JOHN J. MICHON, M.D.

What Is It? · Blepharospasm is a condition in which the muscles in the eyelids and around the eyes twitch uncontrollably. Both eyes are typically affected together, and the spasms usually begin as mild twitches and can progress to forceful blinking. The cause of blepharospasm is unknown. Older patients tend to be affected most often, and women are slightly more prone to the disorder than men. Severe blepharospasm can limit a person's ability to read, drive, or perform other daily activities.

Symptoms: What You May Experience · You may notice frequent, repeated twitching of your eyelids or forceful blinking of both eyes that you cannot control.

Examination Findings: What the Doctor Looks for · Your eye doctor will watch your eyelid movements to determine if blepharospasm is present. He or she will also look for any other causes of excessive blinking, such as dry eye syndrome.

What You Can Do · There is no proven way to avoid the development of blepharospasm. If blepharospasm is causing your eyes to feel irritated, artificial tear drops, lubricating ointment, or both can help.

When to Call the Doctor · If you notice the symptoms of blepharospasm, call your ophthalmologist. Although blepharospasm itself is not dangerous, treating the disorder can make you much more comfortable.

Treatment · The main treatment of blepharospasm is an injection of botulinum toxin (Botox) into the muscles in the eyelids and around the eyes to paralyze them. In the office, your ophthalmologist will inject the botulinum toxin through the skin, using a tiny needle. The botulinum toxin will begin working in about 2–3 days, and its effects typically last for about 3–4 months, after which time the spasms usually reoccur and the botulinum toxin can be injected again. The side effects of botulinum toxin are rare but include droopy eyelids, inability to fully close the eyelids, dry eye, and strabismus.

If botulinum toxin is not effective and the blepharospasm is severe, surgery can be considered. Your ophthalmologist will remove some of the surrounding eye muscles to control the blepharospasm permanently.

Prognosis: Will I See Better? · While blepharospasm is a long-standing disorder, most cases can be treated successfully with botulinum toxin injections. Surgery to remove the muscles, which is rarely needed, is also often successful in reducing the spasms.

http://www.blepharospasm.org/
http://www.ninds.nih.gov/health_and_medical/disorders/
  blepharospasm.htm

6 · Conjunctiva and Sclera

Conjunctivitis (Pink Eye)

SCOTT BLACKMON, M.D.

What Is It? · Conjunctivitis, or "pink eye," is a very common condition characterized by inflammation of the conjunctiva. There are many causes, the most common of which can be grouped into two broad categories: microorganisms (viruses and bacteria, for example) and allergic reactions (medications and pollen, for example). A virus is the most common cause of conjunctivitis.

Symptoms: What You May Experience · Typical symptoms of conjunctivitis include redness of the eyes, tearing or discharge, general discomfort in the eyes, and the feeling that there is "sand" in the eye. In cases of allergic conjunctivitis itching is usually the major complaint, although the other symptoms may also be present.

Examination Findings: What the Doctor Looks for · The most common sign in conjunctivitis is redness over the "whites" of the eyes. There are certain signs that help the eye doctor to determine the cause. For example, does the conjunctivitis involve one or both eyes? Viral or bacterial conjunctivitis usually starts with one eye and may or may not involve the other eye several days later. Is there clear fluid or discharge draining from the eye? Yellow-green discharge suggests that there may be a bacterial cause. Is there enlargement and tenderness of the lymph node just in front of the ear on the same side as the affected eye? This often occurs in viral conjunctivitis. Is there involvement of the cornea? Small areas of corneal involvement may indicate a viral cause and lead to sensitivity to light.

What You Can Do · The most important thing that patients with these symptoms can do is practice good hygiene. Frequent hand washing, keeping the fingers out of the eyes, and not sharing linens are very important to prevent the spread of the contagious forms of conjunctivitis to other people.

When to Call the Doctor · Conjunctivitis accounts for a large number of patient visits to emergency rooms as well as to medicine and eye clinics. It is important to notify your eye doctor if any of the following symptoms are associated with "pink eye": loss of vision, drainage, eye pain, failure to get better within 1–2 weeks, or worsening of symptoms after seeing your doctor.

Treatment · The treatment of conjunctivitis depends on the cause. The most common cause is viral, and the vast majority of cases will heal on their own with no treatment. Therefore, antibiotics are usually not needed to treat "pink eye." Artificial tears and cool compresses may provide symptomatic relief in viral cases. Ophthalmologists may decide to treat with steroid eye drops in some instances, for example if there is corneal involvement associated with reduced vision.

There are certain viruses that do have specific treatment; for example, herpes simplex virus (the same virus responsible for most cold sores) is often treated with antiviral eye drops. If the eye doctor decides that the cause is bacterial, antibiotic eye drops or ointments may be prescribed. There are also eye drops that are effective in treating allergic conjunctivitis. For example, various anti-allergy eye drops and steroid eye drops are often used to provide relief from itching, redness, and other symptoms by inhibiting the eye's immune response. If the symptoms of conjunctivitis are thought to be related to a certain eye medication, the symptoms should subside when the medication is stopped.

Prognosis: Will I See Better? · In uncomplicated cases, patients can expect their symptoms to resolve completely after 1–2 weeks as the conjunctivitis heals. Patients with allergic conjunctivitis can usually find relief from their symptoms with prescription eye drops, although it may take several weeks to find the most effective medication(s). There may also be chronic low-grade symptoms or seasonal flare-ups, especially if the conjunctivitis is related to substances in the air, such as pollen.

www.eyemdlink.com/Condition.asp?ConditionID=6
www.emedicine.com/oph/topic84.htm

Subconjunctival Hemorrhage

SCOTT BLACKMON, M.D.

What Is It? · A subconjunctival hemorrhage is a collection of blood that accumulates under the conjunctiva (the layer over the white of the eyeball) when a small blood vessel bursts. Although most subconjunctival hemorrhages occur in normal, healthy people, patients who have uncontrolled high blood pressure, or who take blood-thinning medications such as aspirin or warfarin, may be more prone to having them.

Symptoms: What You May Experience · You may notice a bright red spot in the normally white part of the eyeball. Occasionally the red spot will look swollen and raised. Your vision is normally not affected. A subconjunctival hemorrhage may cause a feeling of mild eye irritation but should not cause severe eye pain. You may notice a hemorrhage after coughing or straining (due to constipation, for example), or upon awakening.

Examination Findings: What the Doctor Looks for · The eye doctor may see a bright red spot under the conjunctiva. The rest of the eye exam is usually normal.

What You Can Do · Although most subconjunctival hemorrhages occur spontaneously, avoid eye injury, rubbing the eyes, or straining.

When to Call the Doctor · The appearance of a subconjunctival hemorrhage is very striking, prompting many patients to seek medical attention. Usually there is no danger of visual loss. However, these hemorrhages may need immediate attention by an ophthalmologist since they may mask severe injury to the eye. If someone has many recurrent subconjunctival hemorrhages without eye injury or the use of blood thinners, he or she should see a primary medical doctor to check for blood-clotting abnormalities.

Treatment · Artificial tear drops can help with irritation, although these are optional. If a patient is taking a blood-thinning medication, the medication should not be stopped except at the direction of the physician who prescribed it. If someone has many recurrent subconjunctival hemorrhages, clotting studies of the blood and a blood count may be performed.

Prognosis: Will I See Better? · In most cases a subconjunctival hemorrhage is a condition that is not vision-threatening and that will clear up completely in several weeks, with no vision loss or permanent marks left on the eye.

www.emedicine.com/aaem/topic424.htm
www.eyemdlink.com/Condition.asp?ConditionID=127

7 · The Cornea

Dry Eye Syndrome

JULIA SONG, M.D.

What Is It? · Dry eye syndrome is an extremely common condition in which the tear film that lubricates the surface of the eye is abnormal. It is usually due to one of two causes: decreased tear production or increased tear evaporation. Common causes of decreased tear production include Sjogren's syndrome (an autoimmune disorder in which the lacrimal gland is dysfunctional), lacrimal gland disease, and decreased corneal sensation. Common causes of excessive tear evaporation include blepharitis (in which the oil glands around the eyelashes are clogged), blink problems, and eyelid closing problems. Other causes of dry eye syndrome include systemic diseases (sarcoidosis, human immunodeficiency virus [HIV], multiple sclerosis, lymphoma, Stevens-Johnson syndrome, and vitamin A deficiency), certain medications (antihistamines, decongestants, blood pressure medications, and antipsychotic agents), glaucoma eye drops, and prolonged wearing of contact lenses. Postmenopausal women may be especially prone to developing dry eye syndrome. Most cases of dry eye syndrome are not associated with a general medical disease or serious eye problem.

Symptoms: What You May Experience · You may experience a burning sensation in the eye, dryness, the feeling that something is in the eye, blurry vision, and sensitivity to light. These symptoms are often worse at the end of the day or after prolonged use of the eyes.

Examination Findings: What the Doctor Looks for · The eye doctor may see redness or swelling on the white of the eye, decreased tear film, debris in the tear film, an irregular surface of the cornea, or a poor blink response. He or she may put an eye drop in your eyes to check for certain staining patterns on your cornea or conjunctiva. In more severe cases, the doctor may find filaments and mucous plaques. These can be quite painful. In extremely severe cases, your cornea can become thin or, rarely, even perforate.

What You Can Do · You can reduce your chances of dry eyes by avoiding medications that can cause dry eyes, such as antihistamines and decongestants, and by decreasing the amount of time you wear contact lenses.

When to Call the Doctor · If you are experiencing persistent burning and dryness or any decrease in vision, redness, severe pain, or a white spot on the normally clear front surface of your eye, you should contact your eye doctor immediately. Certain causes of dry eyes can lead to an increased risk of infectious keratitis.

Treatment · For mild dry eyes, treatment consists of over-the-counter, preservative-free artificial tear drops, administered up to four times a day, and lubricating ointment at night. If your eyes are moderately dry, you can use preservative-free artificial tear drops up to every hour if needed, as well as ointment at night. Your ophthalmologist may place plugs in your tear ducts so that tears will last longer in your eyes. If you have severe symptoms, you can use these treatments as well as make your environment more moist with a humidifier. Other possibilities include surgery to partially close the eyelid (partial tarsorraphy) or, rarely, a specialized contact lens.

Prognosis: Will I See Better? · Most patients do well with conservative management, such as by using artificial tears and lubricating ointment.

http://www.stlukeseye.com/Conditions/DryEyeSyndrome.asp
http://www.eyemdlink.com/Condition.asp?ConditionID=5

Infectious Keratitis

JULIA SONG, M.D.

What Is It? · Keratitis means inflammation of the cornea. Causes include infection, dry eye syndrome, blepharitis, and autoimmune disorders. Infectious keratitis refers specifically to keratitis caused by a bacterial, viral, or fungal infection. People who wear contact lenses are especially prone to infectious keratitis, and their risk of infection increases as they wear their contact lenses for longer periods. Infectious keratitis can develop into a corneal ulcer if the infection becomes severe.

Symptoms: What You May Experience · You may experience eye pain, redness, decreased vision, and sensitivity to light. The severity of your symptoms may depend on which type of bacterium, virus, or fungus is causing the infection.

Examination Findings: What the Doctor Looks for · The eye doctor looks for infection in the front of the eye with a slit lamp. Signs of infection include redness of the normally clear conjunctiva, whiteness of the normally clear cornea, corneal swelling, abnormal new blood vessels growing in the cornea, and inflammatory cells in the cornea or anterior chamber. The eye doctor may scrape a sample from the surface of the cornea for laboratory evaluation, to determine what type of bacterium, virus, or fungus is causing the infection.

What You Can Do · Avoid eye injury and keep dirt or foreign objects from entering your eyes. Wash your hands thoroughly before touching your eyes or handling contact lenses. Avoid sleeping in contact lenses.

When to Call the Doctor · If you are experiencing any decrease in vision, redness, severe pain, or a white spot on the normally clear front surface of your eye, you should call your eye doctor immediately. Avoid wearing contact lenses if you are having any such eye problems.

Treatment · Treatment depends on the underlying cause of the infectious keratitis. Appropriate antibiotic eye drops, such as antibacterial, antiviral, or antifungal agents, will likely be prescribed for frequent use (as often as every 30 to 60 minutes in severe infections). In certain cases, oral antibiotics can also help treat the infection.

Prognosis: Will I See Better? · Vision often improves with treatment of the underlying infection. However, there may be some scarring of the cornea after treatment that may or may not affect vision in the long run. If the corneal scarring is in the center of the cornea, where it affects the line of sight, a corneal transplant may ultimately be needed to improve the vision.

http://www.intelihealth.com/IH/ihtIH/WSIHW000/9339/9942.html
http://www.nlm.nih.gov/medlineplus/ency/article/001032.htm

Corneal Abrasion

JULIA SONG, M.D.

What Is It? · A corneal abrasion is a scratch on the cornea (the clear, nonwhite surface of the eye). An abrasion can be caused by an eye injury (such as from a fingernail, a paper cut, a foreign body, or a contact lens).

Symptoms: What You May Experience · You may have immediate pain, the feeling that something is in your eye, tearing, or discomfort with blinking.

Examination Findings: What the Doctor Looks for · Your doctor may use an eye drop that has a special dye to see an area of staining where the top layer, or epithelium, of the cornea is missing. He or she may also see redness and inflammation of your eye.

What You Can Do · Avoid injury to your eyes. Decrease the length of time you wear your contact lenses.

When to Call the Doctor · If you are experiencing any decrease in vision, redness, severe pain, or a white spot on the normally clear front surface of your eye, you should contact your ophthalmologist immediately.

Treatment · Treatment usually depends on the size and cause of the abrasion. If it is small, it can be treated with antibiotic eye drops or ointment. If it is larger, antibiotic drops, certain dilating drops (cycloplegics), and rarely pressure patching may be needed.

If organic material (such as grass, plants, or wood) is the cause of the abrasion, then the abrasion is considered dirty and the eye will need to be examined more frequently for possible secondary infection. No pressure patching is recommended for abrasions caused by organic material or contact lenses.

Prognosis: Will I See Better? · Corneal abrasions generally heal in several days, with vision returning to normal. A secondary infection may make treatment more difficult. In patients with diabetes mellitus, a corneal abrasion heals more slowly.

http://www.emedicine.com/EMERG/topic828.htm
http://www.eyemdlink.com/Condition.asp?ConditionID=141

Recurrent Corneal Erosion Syndrome

JULIA SONG, M.D.

What Is It? · This syndrome consists of recurrent corneal abrasions due to a loose top layer of the cornea called the epithelium. There may be a history of a corneal abrasion that occurred weeks, months, or years before the current episode. During the healing process, the corneal epithelium does not bind well to its underlying membrane and remains somewhat looser than normal, making future abrasions more likely. Patients with corneal epithelial basement membrane dystrophies are at risk for developing recurrent corneal erosions spontaneously or with mild trauma. Other predisposing conditions include meibomian gland dysfunction (clogged oil glands around the eyelashes), diabetes, prior corneal infection, other corneal dystrophies, or refractive surgery (LASIK).

Symptoms: What You May Experience · You may experience the feeling that something is in your eye, intense eye pain, or tearing. These symptoms often occur upon awakening.

Examination Findings: What the Doctor Looks for · Your eye doctor may use a yellow eye drop to see an area of green staining on the cornea using a blue light, where the epithelium of the cornea is missing. He or she may find that the top layer of the cornea looks rough and irregular. If the cause is a corneal epithelial basement membrane dystrophy, your doctor may see corneal abnormalities in your other eye.

What You Can Do · Avoid trauma if possible and minimize rubbing of the eye.

When to Call the Doctor · If you experience any decrease in vision, redness, severe pain, or a white spot on the front clear surface of your eye, you should contact your eye doctor immediately.

Treatment · Conservative management for acute recurrent erosions often consists of frequent lubrication with antibiotic ointment. Hypertonic saline (5% sodium chloride) eye drops can also be used. In more severe cases, your eye doctor may prescribe a bandage contact lens. If there is associated inflammation, he or she may add steroid eye drops.

If conservative management does not work, anterior stromal puncture may be performed in certain cases, such as recurrent erosion syndrome that occurs after eye injury but is not in the central zone of the cornea. In this technique, your eye doctor makes tiny puncture marks in the affected areas with a needle, so the top layer of the cornea will heal and stick more tightly to its basement membrane. This is done in the clinic. Another treatment option is epithelial debridement, which involves peeling off the corneal epithelium. A bandage contact lens is used for several days afterward, until the epithelium regenerates. Laser (phototherapeutic keratectomy) has been found useful in rare cases.

Prognosis: Will I See Better? · Vision often returns to normal when the erosion has healed. A secondary infection may limit visual recovery. In some cases there may be scarring of the cornea after treatment that may affect visual recovery.

http://www.stlukeseye.com/Conditions/CornealErosion.asp
http://www.emedicine.com/oph/topic113.htm

Corneal Ulcer

ROSANNA P. BAHADUR, M.D. · NATALIE A. AFSHARI, M.D.

What Is It? · A corneal ulcer is a deep infection in the cornea, the clear, front surface of the eye. The infection usually develops from wearing contact lenses or after the cornea is scratched by an object such as a fingernail (a corneal abrasion). The type of organism causing the infection is usually a bacterium or fungus. Corneal ulcers can be very aggressive and harmful if not found early and treated appropriately by an eye doctor.

Symptoms: What You May Experience · If you develop a corneal ulcer, you may notice a decrease in your vision, tearing, milky or colored eye discharge, eye pain or redness, or sensitivity to light. You may see a white spot on the normally clear cornea.

Examination Findings: What the Doctor Looks for · Your doctor will examine your cornea with a slit lamp to look for a scratch with infection beneath it. He or she will also look for infection and inflammation in the tissues surrounding the cornea and in the anterior chamber. If a corneal ulcer is large or located in the center of the cornea, your eye doctor may perform cultures to identify the specific bacterium or fungus causing the infection. The ulcer will be measured so that its size and progress can be followed from visit to visit.

What You Can Do · Use eye protection and avoid eye rubbing to prevent a corneal abrasion. If you think you may have scratched your eye, remove your contact lenses. Avoid sleeping in contact lenses, and never use tap water or saliva to clean your lenses.

When to Call the Doctor · If you think your eye may be scratched or if you develop vision loss, tearing, milky or colored eye discharge, eye pain or redness, or sensitivity to light, call your eye doctor promptly.

Treatment · Your eye doctor may prescribe antibiotic eye drops to target the bacterium or fungus causing the infection. These antibiotic eye drops may need to be used as often as every 30 minutes.

He or she may also prescribe a dilating eye drop to decrease inflammation. You will likely have frequent eye exams while the corneal ulcer is being treated. If the ulcer causes significant corneal scarring after it has healed, a corneal transplant may ultimately be necessary in rare cases.

Prognosis: Will I See Better? · Many people have improved vision after a corneal ulcer has healed. In cases where serious scarring of the cornea results, the vision may be poor unless a corneal transplant is performed.

http://www.nei.nih.gov/health/cornealdisease/index.htm#3
http://www.nlm.nih.gov/medlineplus/ency/article/001032.htm

Keratoconus

ROSANNA P. BAHADUR, M.D. · NATALIE A. AFSHARI, M.D.

What Is It? · The cornea is the clear, dome-shaped surface that covers the front central area of the eyeball and focuses light on the retina. In keratoconus the cornea is abnormally shaped because its middle area is thin and bulges out, resulting in a cone shape rather than a smoothly curved cornea. Mild cases may cause distorted vision because of the cornea's shape. In moderate or severe keratoconus, the thinned cornea can develop tiny cracks that lead to corneal swelling and eye pain (acute hydrops). Scarring of the cornea can also occur.

In the United States keratoconus occurs in about 1 of every 2,000 people, most of whom are diagnosed in their teens or early twenties. The shape of the cornea in keratoconus tends to stabilize after young adulthood. When present, keratoconus is almost always found in both eyes, but one eye may be worse than the other. The cause of the disease is not known, but keratoconus can run in families and has been linked to frequent eye rubbing, long-term use of contact lenses, Down syndrome, and other rare diseases.

Symptoms: What You May Experience · You may have trouble seeing clearly even with a new eyeglass prescription, and your prescription may change significantly between regular eye exams. If you wear contact lenses, the lenses may easily fall out of your eyes.

Examination Findings: What the Doctor Looks for · The eye doctor will examine the shape of your cornea with a slit lamp and look for thin or steep areas. Specialized photographs of the cornea called corneal topography may be taken to measure the cornea's steepness and shape.

What You Can Do · Reduce the number of hours you wear contact lenses and avoid rubbing your eyes excessively. Keeping up with regular eye exams can help your eye doctor notice if your glasses prescription changes rapidly.

When to Call the Doctor · If you notice decreased vision despite a new eyeglass prescription, you should call your eye doctor. If you have keratoconus and experience eye pain, excessive tearing, or decreased vision, call your eye doctor, since these symptoms could mean that your cornea has thinned to a certain point and needs treatment.

Treatment · In mild keratoconus, properly prescribed eyeglasses or, more commonly, hard contact lenses usually improve vision by compensating for the steepness of the cornea. Episodes of acute hydrops may be treated with eye drops or a soft contact lens. In moderate or severe keratoconus, a corneal transplant may ultimately be needed.

Prognosis: Will I See Better? · Most keratoconus patients do extremely well with hard contact lenses. If corneal transplantation is necessary, these patients tend to heal well, and many experience good vision afterward.

www.nkcf.org **http:**//www.kcenter.org/index.html

Corneal Transplant

ROSANNA P. BAHADUR, M.D. · NATALIE A. AFSHARI, M.D.
When a normally clear cornea becomes cloudy, it blocks light from reaching the retina. If this happens to you, you and your

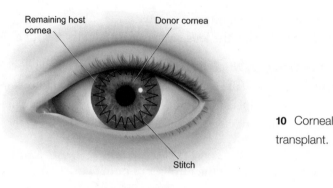

Remaining host cornea

Donor cornea

Stitch

10 Corneal transplant.

ophthalmologist may decide that a corneal transplant is needed to improve your vision. A corneal transplant is a surgery in which a diseased cornea is replaced with a clear, healthy, donor cornea. Donor corneas come from people who have agreed to donate their eye tissue after they die to help others regain their sight.

After a donor dies, the corneas are removed and taken to an eye bank, where they are examined to make sure that they are healthy. The cornea is a unique tissue, because unlike other transplanted organs it does not have to be matched to the patient receiving the transplant. The eye bank keeps the donor corneas until they are needed for corneal transplant surgery.

Corneal transplantation is an outpatient surgery performed in the operating room. Most patients are given intravenous sedation and numbing medicine is placed around the eye so that the operation is painless. The diseased cornea is removed using an instrument called a trephine that resembles a cookie cutter. A healthy donor cornea is cut to fit, and then sewn in place using microscopic sutures. This procedure usually takes 60–90 minutes, followed by a short recovery time.

After surgery, your cornea surgeon will check your eye the next day. He or she will prescribe antibiotic and steroid eye drops to be used while the transplant heals. Normal activities can be resumed after corneal transplantation with some limitations. Heavy lifting, bending, or straining should be avoided after surgery until approved by your surgeon. Some form of eye protection should be worn at all times after surgery to protect the transplant and the tiny stitches holding it in place. It is normal to feel some scratchiness and eye irritation shortly after the surgery.

The improvement in vision after a corneal transplant is different for each patient, but achieving this best possible vision usually takes 6–12 months. At each follow-up exam your cornea surgeon may remove some of the stitches, which is a painless procedure performed in the office, to reduce astigmatism in the transplant. Some patients achieve their best vision after a corneal transplant by wearing a hard contact lens over the transplanted cornea. You will likely need to use a steroid eye drop long term to help prevent your body from rejecting the transplanted cornea and causing it to fail.

As with all surgeries, there are risks and benefits of corneal transplantation that your ophthalmologist will discuss with you. After surgery, using the recommended eye drops and keeping up with scheduled follow-up exams will give your new cornea the best chance to improve your vision.

http://www.eyebank.org/corneal.html
http://www.nlm.nih.gov/medlineplus/ency/article/003008.htm

Cataract

TERRY SEMCHYSHYN, M.D.

What Is It? · A cataract is a natural clouding of the normally clear lens inside the eye that occurs with age. Light must pass through the lens to reach the retina, and a cataract makes the vision hazy. Cataracts are part of the natural aging process and are found in over 75% of people over the age of 70. The lens is clear at birth, but with time it becomes hazier and more yellow or brown. Cataracts are one of the most common causes of treatable, reversible vision loss.

The most common type of cataract is an age-related cataract. Much less commonly, cataracts can be present at birth; these are called congenital cataracts. A cataract that forms as a result of an eye injury is a traumatic cataract. Certain medical conditions (such as diabetes) and certain medicines (such as steroids) can cause cataracts to become cloudy at a faster rate. However, it is impossible to predict how quickly a cataract will progress.

In most cases, cataracts do not cause permanent damage to the eye besides affecting the vision. However, rare cases of extremely advanced cataracts may result in inflammation or high eye pressure.

Symptoms: What You May Experience · Your vision may gradually become blurred over months or years and you may notice sensitivity to light or glare. Poor night vision, difficulty driving, and needing brighter light to read are common symptoms of cataracts. Some people also experience double vision in one eye, fading or yellowing of colors, or frequent eyeglass prescription changes, especially after years of stable vision. Cataracts may cause some people to no longer need their eyeglasses as the cataract changes the way the eye refracts, or bends, light (known as "second sight").

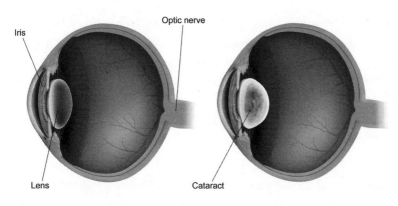

Iris

Optic nerve

Lens

Cataract

11 Left: normal lens. Right: cataract lens.

Cataracts are so named (the word means "waterfall") because having a cataract may give the impression of looking through the mist or fog from a waterfall. Cataracts are typically painless.

Examination Findings: What the Doctor Looks for · Your eye doctor will notice that your vision may be blurred even with the best glasses prescription. Your doctor may also perform a "glare test" by shining bright lights toward your eyes while you read the eye chart. This test simulates glare from sunshine or car headlights. Your doctor may dilate your pupils to see the lens better with a microscope. He or she will also look for other possible causes of your blurry vision.

What You Can Do · There are no known medicines, vitamin supplements, or exercises that can prevent or cure cataracts. Protection from excess ultraviolet (uv) light with sunglasses may help slow the progression of cataracts.

When to Call the Doctor · If you start to notice painless blurry vision, glare, sensitivity to light, or poor vision in dim light, you should make an appointment with your eye doctor. Cataracts do not harm the eye in most cases, but they do cause your vision to become blurrier over time. Trouble driving, especially at night, and having to use brighter lights to read comfortably are other reasons to call your eye doctor.

Treatment · Cataract surgery should be considered when the cataract causes enough blurriness to interfere with your daily activities. Surgery is the only known way to treat cataracts. It can improve vision and make colors seem brighter. If a cataract makes your vision only slightly blurry, then a follow-up visit in several months or a year may be recommended before it is decided whether surgery is needed.

Prognosis: Will I See Better? · Cataract surgery is one of the most common and most successful surgeries performed in the United States today. If a cataract is the main cause of blurry vision, then your chance of seeing better after cataract surgery is quite good.

http://www.aao.org
http://www.nei.nih.gov/health/cataract/cataract_facts.asp

Cataract Surgery

TERRY SEMCHYSHYN, M.D.

What Is It? · Once your eye doctor has diagnosed a cataract that is affecting your vision, using surgery to remove the cloudy lens is the only way to treat it. In small-incision surgery, a very small opening (1/8th of an inch) is made in the eye, and an ultrasound instrument breaks the cataract into small pieces and then removes them (phacoemulsification). Often a permanent, clear, artificial lens implant is then inserted inside the eye in place of the natural lens to help focus light. A stitch may or may not be used to close the small opening in the eye at the end of the operation. Your eye surgeon performs this extremely delicate surgery with a powerful magnifying microscope.

What You May Experience · Once you and your doctor have decided to have your cataract removed, your eye will be measured in the office for the new artificial lens implant. Your surgery will usually be an outpatient or same-day surgery, meaning that if your surgery goes well, you will come to the hospital the day of the surgery and go home after the operation on the same day.

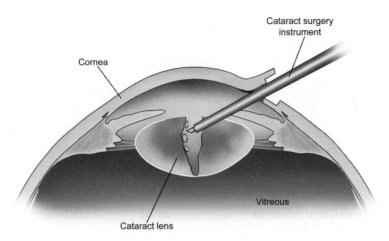

Cataract surgery
instrument

Cornea

Vitreous

Cataract lens

12 Instrument placed in eyeball for cataract surgery.

You will be asked not to eat or drink after midnight the night be-fore your surgery to avoid having an upset stomach during your surgery.

Most patients are not put completely to sleep (general anesthe-sia) for cataract surgery, but instead may be given intravenous sedation to relax, as well as numbing eye drops or a numbing in-jection around the eye. During the surgery, you may hear your surgeon speak or the sound of instruments working, and you may see bright lights and changing colors, but you will not see the de-tails of the actual surgery. Near the end of your surgery, the micro-scope light may become very bright as your lens implant is fitted inside your eye. Once the surgery is over, your doctor may put a small shield over your eye to protect it.

After visiting the recovery area and having something to eat or drink, you are usually able to go home. You will be asked to use eye drops after your surgery. Your eye doctor will usually see you in the office the next morning and several times afterward. You will likely need a new glasses prescription several weeks after surgery.

If you have cataracts in both eyes, only one eye is treated at a time; usually the second cataract can be removed several months after the first.

Examination Findings: What the Doctor Looks for · During your eye exams after cataract surgery, your eye doctor checks for inflammation, infection, and proper position of the lens implant.

What You Can Do · Make sure you take all medicines and eye drops as directed. After surgery, your doctor may ask you to wear glasses during the day and an eye shield while sleeping to protect your eye. Avoid dusty or dirty areas, and do not bend over at the waist. Ask your doctor when you can return to driving and your usual physical activity.

When to Call the Doctor · While cataract surgery usually goes very well, every surgery has risks of complications. Possible complications of cataract surgery include bleeding, infection, needing further surgery, a poor cosmetic result, retinal detachment, high eye pressure, and, extremely rarely, even loss of vision or of the eye itself. After surgery, you should call your eye doctor immediately if your vision worsens, if you have eye pain not relieved by over-the-counter pain medication, if you vomit, if you injure your eye, or if anything seems worse.

Prognosis: Will I See Better? · Cataract surgery is one of the more successful surgeries performed today, and visual improvement is often excellent. Sometimes other eye problems, such as glaucoma, diabetic retinopathy, or macular degeneration, can limit your potential vision. However, even with such limits, cataract surgery can still help make your vision brighter or improve your side vision.

http://www.aao.org
http://www.nei.nih.gov/health/cataract/cataract_facts.asp

Posterior Capsule Opacification ("After Cataract")

TERRY SEMCHYSHYN, M.D.

What Is It? · In many cases after cataract surgery, a thin film or haze, called a posterior capsular opacity or "after cataract," can form behind the lens implant. This film is caused by remaining microscopic lens cells that continue to grow on the naturally clear capsule that holds the lens implant in place. Usually this haze develops a few months after cataract surgery. It is painless and harmless to the eye but causes the vision to become more blurred over time. A new glasses prescription will not improve vision in these cases because the light must still travel through the haze to get into the eye.

About 50% of the people who develop a posterior capsular opacity will need laser treatment to improve their vision. The laser helps to make an opening in this haze, which is sized to fit the patient's pupil, so light can travel clearly into the eye. After this haze is treated by laser, it does not grow back.

Symptoms: What You May Experience · Your vision may slowly become blurry over the months following cataract surgery. You may notice glare with bright lights at night, and in fact you may have changes in your vision similar to those that you experienced while you still had your original cataract.

Examination Findings: What the Doctor Looks for · Your eye doctor may be able to detect a posterior capsular opacity during your visits after surgery. He or she will see a hazy film on the capsule behind your lens implant. If your eye doctor thinks the film is thick enough to affect your vision, he or she may recommend laser treatment.

What You Can Do · There is no way for you to prevent a posterior capsular opacity from forming.

When to Call the Doctor · You should call your eye doctor if you notice your vision getting hazier and blurrier after cataract surgery. If you have recently had the laser treatment and you notice flashing lights, many new floaters, or a black curtain in your vision, call your ophthalmologist immediately. These changes could be warning signs of a retinal detachment that needs urgent treatment.

Treatment · The laser treatment is usually done in your ophthalmologist's office and does not require a visit to the operating room. Your ophthalmologist may use a special contact lens on your eye to help guide the laser. The treatment itself normally takes several minutes. Afterward your eye doctor may check your eye pressure and ask you to use steroid eye drops for a few days to suppress any inflammation from the laser.

In general, laser treatment for a posterior capsular opacity is low risk. However, rare complications from the laser include high eye pressure, inflammation, retinal detachment, and dislocation of the lens implant.

Prognosis: Will I See Better? · Posterior capsular opacities can generally be treated very well with laser surgery, often improving vision back to its original level after the cataract surgery.

http://www.aao.org
http://www.eyemdlink.com/Condition.asp?ConditionID=354

Dislocated Lens

TERRY SEMCHYSHYN, M.D.

What Is It? · Dislocation of either a natural lens or a lens implant after cataract surgery means that the lens shifts from its proper position within the eye. If the shift is large enough, it can cause blurry vision, similar to how the vision might change if your glasses slid down to the tip of your nose. Dislocation of a natural lens can happen after eye injury or spontaneously because of certain medical conditions.

Dislocation of a lens implant after cataract surgery can also occur. During cataract surgery, a permanent artificial lens implant is often placed in the eye to improve vision. The lens implant is usually supported by the same capsular bag that gave support to the original natural lens. This bag normally supports the lens implant adequately, but it can shift or develop openings that can cause the lens implant inside it to shift.

A lens or lens implant that shifts but stays within the capsular bag is called a subluxed lens. A dislocated lens, on the other hand, occurs if the lens or lens implant moves out of the bag, or if both the bag and the lens move away from their normal positions. Both subluxation and dislocation of a lens or lens implant can cause blurry vision.

Symptoms: What You May Experience · You may experience blurry vision or double vision, both of which may worsen over time. Wearing glasses does not usually improve the vision.

Examination Findings: What the Doctor Looks for · Your eye doctor will check the position of your lens or lens implant using a slit lamp.

What You Can Do · The only way you can prevent lens dislocation is to avoid eye injury. Follow your doctor's instructions about eye protection after cataract surgery.

When to Call the Doctor · Call your eye doctor if you have double vision that is not improved by your glasses or if your vision suddenly becomes worse.

Treatment · A lens or lens implant that is only slightly out of position may not affect your vision enough to need treatment. A subluxed or dislocated natural lens may need to be removed with surgery. A subluxed or dislocated lens implant may be put back in its proper location with surgery or possibly exchanged with a lens implant that can be anchored differently to the eye.

Prognosis: Will I See Better? · Often surgery for lens dislocation is quite successful in improving vision. Rarely the dislocated lens or lens implant may damage the retina or other important parts inside the eye, ultimately limiting your vision.

http://www.aao.org
http://www.intelihealth.com/IH/ihtIH/WSIHW000/9339/9933.html

Age-Related Macular Degeneration

SRILAXMI BEARELLY, M.D. · MICHAEL J. COONEY, M.D.

What Is It? · Age-related macular degeneration (AMD) is the leading cause of central vision loss in the western world in people over
the age of 55. AMD is an age-associated degenerative disorder of the
macula, which is the portion of the retina responsible for central
vision. In AMD the cells that make up the macula become damaged, resulting in central vision loss.

There are a number of reasons why people may develop AMD,
including increasing age, genetic and hereditary factors, and en-
vironmental risk factors. Since pigment in the eyes appears to
be protective, Caucasians, particularly women, appear to be at
greater risk. Smoking, family history, nutrition, and sunlight exposure over the course of one's lifetime may also play a role.

There are two forms of AMD, a more common dry form and a
less common wet form. In the dry form, which affects 90% of AMD
patients, aging deposits called drusen become deposited underneath the macula. In the vast majority of patients, these drusen
cause no visual changes; however, in some the drusen can cause
the macula to thin, resulting in a slow, gradual decrease in central vision. If the drusen cause substantial weakening of important
layers in the macula, the wet form of AMD may then develop.

Wet AMD develops when abnormal blood vessels start to grow
through the layers of the macula that have been weakened by the
dry form of AMD. These abnormal blood vessels can cause bleeding, leakage of fluid, and the formation of scar tissue, which in
turn can lead to a rapid and severe loss of central vision.

Although only 1 in 10 patients with AMD will convert from the
dry to the wet form, the wet form accounts for 90% of the vision
loss associated with AMD. The chance of a patient with dry AMD

converting to the more aggressive wet form is approximately 2% each year.

Symptoms: What You May Experience · The vast majority of patients with dry AMD will not notice any changes in their central vision. However, patients with advanced dry AMD may notice a gradual decrease in their central vision, as well as formation of a central blind spot over many months to years. The most common symptom of wet AMD is the sudden onset of blurred or distorted central vision that may occur over days to weeks. AMD is painless.

Examination Findings: What the Doctor Looks for · After checking your vision and performing a routine eye exam, the eye doctor will dilate your eyes to obtain a view of the macula so that he or she can look for signs of AMD. If wet AMD is suspected, a fluorescein angiogram (photographic dye test) may be obtained. In some cases, optical coherence tomography (OCT), another photographic test, may be performed as well.

What You Can Do · There is currently no proven way to prevent AMD, although avoiding smoking and maintaining a healthy diet may help reduce the risk of developing the disease. Because AMD is a relatively silent disease until the advanced stages develop, all patients over the age of 55 should have an annual dilated eye examination to look for early signs of AMD. Now that treatments are available for most patients with either the dry or the wet form, it is important that AMD be diagnosed as early as possible so that appropriate treatment can be started promptly. If you have AMD, regular home use of an Amsler grid (which your eye doctor may provide) can help you monitor changes in your central vision.

When to Call the Doctor · If you notice blurry or decreased central vision, you should call your eye doctor. If you have known AMD and you notice changes in your central vision, you should see your eye doctor promptly.

Treatment · The Age-Related Eye Disease Study (AREDS), a ten-year study sponsored by the National Eye Institute, found that a high-dose supplement of antioxidants and zinc significantly de-

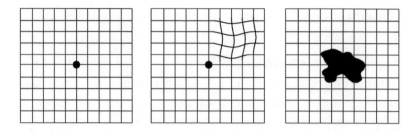

13 Left: normal Amsler grid. Center: distorted Amsler grid. Right: blind spot in center of Amsler grid.

creased the progression and vision loss associated with AMD. The formula was also proven to reduce the chance of conversion from the dry to the wet form among patients with advanced AMD. This formula includes daily intake of vitamin C (500 mg), vitamin E (400 IU), beta-carotene (15 mg), zinc oxide (80 mg), and cupric oxide (2 mg). Some patients with AMD, especially present and past smokers, should not be on these vitamins; thus, patients must discuss vitamin supplementation with their medical doctors. Supplemental beta carotene in particular should be avoided by all smokers.

There are several types of treatment for wet AMD, all of which are designed to contain the growth of abnormal blood vessels underneath the retina to stabilize the vision. One treatment involves a conventional thermal, or hot, laser, which cauterizes the abnormal blood vessels. Another is photodynamic therapy, which uses a drug called verteporfin that is injected intravenously. The drug is then activated by a special laser which causes the blood vessels to close. Surgical methods of treatment include macular translocation, which moves the macula away from the abnormal blood vessels onto a new location of healthier tissue. Patients may be candidates for one or another of these treatments depending on several factors, including the type and location of blood vessels.

Areas of current research include anti-angiogenesis medications such as Macugen injected into the eyeball (to stop the growth of blood vessels), forms of laser therapy such as transpupillary thermotherapy and feeder vessel therapy, and surgeries such as submacular surgery and retinal cell transplantation.

Prognosis: Will I See Better? · Most patients with AMD do not experience vision loss. For those with decreased vision from AMD, the disease usually does not improve over time, though in some cases it can stabilize on its own. Many currently available AMD treatments are designed to preserve the central vision rather than improve it.

Although AMD can significantly challenge one's central vision, it is important for patients with AMD to know that this disease almost always only affects central vision and almost never will cause them to go "completely blind." In fact, in 99% of cases the peripheral, or side, vision remains unaffected, allowing for independent living.

www.amdcenter.org **http:**//www.nei.nih.gov/amd/pr.htm

Central Serous Chorioretinopathy

DAVID YEH, M.D.

What Is It? · Central serous chorioretinopathy (CSCR) is a condition in which fluid leaks and accumulates under the macula, the central part of the retina. Although anyone can be affected, it typically occurs between the ages of 20 and 50, and is up to 10 times more common in males. The cause of CSCR is unknown, but there have been some associations with stress ("type A personality"), high blood pressure, pregnancy, and the use of steroid medications. In most cases the fluid is spontaneously reabsorbed slowly over weeks to months, and the vision improves.

Usually only one eye is affected. However, CSCR can recur in the same eye or the other eye. Rarely, CSCR may result in choroidal neovascularization, a more serious condition in which abnormal blood vessels grow under the retina.

Symptoms: What You May Experience · You may notice the sudden onset of painless, blurry vision or a blind spot in the center of your vision. Other symptoms include visual distortion (objects may seem smaller than usual or straight lines may appear wavy) and decreased color brightness.

Examination Findings: What the Doctor Looks for · A careful retinal exam by your eye doctor will often reveal the leaked fluid. A photographic dye test called fluorescein angiography and optical coherence tomography may also be performed to confirm the diagnosis of CSCR and rule out other diseases.

What You Can Do · There is little you can do to prevent CSCR or hasten its resolution. Although attempting to reduce your stress level may help, there is no proven benefit to addressing this or other risk factors. If you are using inhaled or systemic steroid medication, check with your medical doctor to see if another medication could be substituted for the steroid.

When to Call the Doctor · If you experience vision loss or distortion, you should contact your eye doctor. Although CSCR may be the cause, there are many other potentially serious causes of visual loss or distortion.

Treatment · CSCR usually resolves on its own and does not require specific treatment. In certain cases, hot laser treatment performed in the clinic may speed recovery. However, laser treatment has potential risks and does not change the final visual outcome. Photodynamic therapy may be another treatment option in some cases.

Prognosis: Will I See Better? · In 80–90% of cases, a full or nearly full recovery occurs over about 6 months, although some mild residual symptoms may be expected. A small number of people will have multiple recurrences, which may lead to permanent visual loss over time.

http://www.emedicine.com/oph/topic689.htm
http://www.stlukeseye.com/Conditions/CSCR.asp

Cystoid Macular Edema

DAVID YEH, M.D.

What Is It? · Cystoid macular edema (CME) refers to fluid leakage into the macula, the central part of the retina. The fluid collects in small pockets (called cysts) within the retina, which causes swelling that can affect vision. CME is not a single disease, but rather a way that the retina responds to a variety of diseases. It is a common cause of decreased vision after cataract surgery, but it may also result from other eye conditions such as diabetes, retinal vein occlusions, inflammation (uveitis), and other eye surgeries.

Symptoms: What You May Experience · You may notice a gradual, painless decrease in vision, distortion in vision (e.g., straight lines may appear wavy), or alterations in color vision. In CME after cataract surgery, patients typically describe improved vision after the surgery, followed by a gradual deterioration several weeks later.

Examination Findings: What the Doctor Looks for · A careful retinal exam by your eye doctor may reveal the fluid-filled cysts and swelling. Often additional photographic tests such as fluorescein angiography or optical coherence tomography are needed to confirm the diagnosis. The doctor will also look for signs of other eye diseases which might be causing CME.

What You Can Do · In most cases there is little you can do to prevent CME or hasten its resolution directly. Taking care of specific diseases such as diabetes and following your doctor's advice regarding these diseases is important.

When to Call the Doctor · If you experience decreased or distorted vision, you should contact your eye doctor. Although CME may be the cause, there are many other potentially serious causes of visual loss or distortion.

Treatment · CME can be treated in various ways, depending on its cause. After eye surgery, eye drops such as steroids and other anti-inflammatory medications are often used. In other cases laser treatment may be recommended. Other forms of steroids, including those taken by mouth or injected into or around the eye, are sometimes used. Finally, some cases may require specialized eye surgery (vitrectomy).

Prognosis: Will I See Better? · Visual prognosis for CME depends on the cause and severity. CME following cataract surgery has an excellent chance of improving on its own or with medications. CME from other causes has a variable outcome, although some visual improvement can usually be expected. The improvement is often gradual over the course of several months. Long-standing CME can sometimes lead to permanent visual loss, which may not improve even after the CME disappears.

http://www.emedicine.com/oph/topic400.htm
http://www.emedicine.com/oph/topic638.htm

Diabetic Retinopathy

DAVID YEH, M.D.

What Is It? · Diabetic retinopathy is an eye disease caused by diabetes mellitus. Diabetes inflicts damage on blood vessels all over the body, including in the eye. In the United States diabetic retinopathy is the leading cause of acquired blindness between the ages of 25 and 74.

Type 1 (insulin-dependent) as well as type 2 (non-insulin-dependent) diabetics of any age can develop diabetic retinopathy. Risk factors for developing diabetic retinopathy include having diabetes for a long time and poor blood sugar control. Although progression of the disease is highly variable, most people who have had diabetes for at least 20 years have some degree of diabetic retinopathy.

Diabetic retinopathy is divided into non-proliferative (or "background") and proliferative forms. Non-proliferative diabetic retinopathy develops first and is characterized by small areas of bleeding and fluid leakage from damaged blood vessels. Often patients with the non-proliferative form do not have visual symptoms. However, non-proliferative diabetic retinopathy may cause reduc-

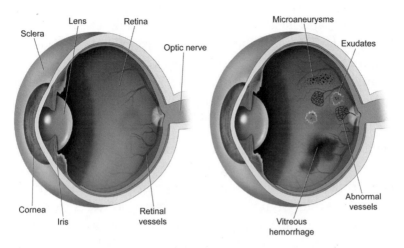

14 Left: normal retina. Right: retina affected by diabetic retinopathy.

tion of blood flow to the retina (known as macular ischemia), and excessive leakage can cause swelling of the retina (called diabetic macular edema), both of which may affect vision. Proliferative diabetic retinopathy is more threatening and is characterized by the growth of new abnormal blood vessels in the eye as the body attempts to increase blood flow to the retina. These new blood vessels are abnormally fragile and can bleed easily (causing a vitreous hemorrhage when the eye fills with blood). Retinal scarring, retinal detachment, and severe glaucoma can also develop and lead to serious vision loss.

Symptoms: What You May Experience · In the early stages of diabetic retinopathy, you may not notice any visual changes. As the disease progresses, you may notice blurry vision, which may be gradual or sudden. A vitreous hemorrhage may appear as sudden vision loss with floaters. Retinal detachments may be accompanied by flashes and floaters as well. There is usually no pain in diabetic retinopathy, except when glaucoma caused by severe proliferative diabetic retinopathy leads to very high eye pressures.

Examination Findings: What the Doctor Looks for · During the exam the eye doctor looks for retinal bleeding and swelling, retinal detachments, and glaucoma. Photographs of the retina may also be taken to document the level of disease for future reference. Fluorescein angiography, a photographic dye test, can help to evaluate blood flow to the retina and identify abnormal leakage. In some cases, optical coherence tomography (another photographic test) may also be performed.

What You Can Do · In addition to getting regular eye exams, the best treatment for preventing or slowing the progression of diabetic retinopathy is to carefully control your blood sugar. This requires close collaboration with your primary medical doctor, with regular monitoring and adjustment of medications as needed. You should keep records of your blood sugar levels and your most recent hemoglobin A1C blood test result (which is a three-month average of your blood sugar levels) for your eye doctor to review. In addition to blood sugar control, you should also be checked for high blood pressure and high cholesterol, which should also be optimally controlled.

When to Call the Doctor · All diabetic patients should receive regular eye exams. Depending on the severity of disease, these may be scheduled anywhere from once yearly to once every few months. In addition, if you experience worsening vision, sudden visual loss, flashes, floaters, or eye pain, you should contact your eye doctor, who may wish to see you sooner.

Treatment · The treatment of diabetic retinopathy depends on the severity of disease and the specific complications that arise. Nonproliferative diabetic retinopathy, unless severe, usually requires only regular monitoring. Laser treatment may be performed for both diabetic macular edema (to reduce swelling) and for proliferative diabetic retinopathy (to cause regression of the abnormal blood vessels). Glaucoma may require the use of pressure-lowering eye drops. Surgical treatment is usually reserved for the most severe complications, such as severe vitreous hemorrhage, retinal detachment, or severe glaucoma. Newer treatments continue to be developed, including steroid injections into the eye for macular edema unresponsive to laser.

Prognosis: Will I See Better? · When diabetic retinopathy results in visual loss, improvement in vision depends on the severity of the disease and the specific complication causing the visual loss. If the vision loss is from vitreous hemorrhage, it may improve as the blood is reabsorbed or surgically removed. Surgical repair of retinal detachments may also result in visual improvement. In many cases, however, vision loss from diabetes is permanent, and the goal of treatment is not to restore lost vision but rather to prevent or slow further visual loss. Some treatments may even worsen certain parts of the vision in an attempt to preserve central vision. Therefore, prevention remains the key to controlling diabetic retinopathy.

http://www.emedicine.com/oph/topic414.htm
http://www.emedicine.com/oph/topic415.htm

Endophthalmitis

MILA OH, M.D.

What Is It? · Endophthalmitis is a rare but serious infection inside the eyeball, usually caused by bacteria. Most cases of endophthalmitis occur within 1 to 14 days after cataract surgery or other eye surgery, but endophthalmitis can also occur months or years later in certain cases, especially after glaucoma surgery. Rarely, endophthalmitis is caused by eye injury or by infections that spread to the eye from other parts of the body.

Symptoms: What You May Experience · Symptoms include decreasing vision, severe eye pain, and redness, all of which may develop rapidly.

Examination Findings: What the Doctor Looks for · Your eye doctor will check your vision and eye pressure. Your pupil will be dilated so that your eye doctor can look for signs of infection inside your eye. In some cases, an ultrasound of the eyeball may be performed.

What You Can Do · Although there is nothing known to prevent endophthalmitis, good hygienic practices such as washing your hands with clean water before touching your eyes and keeping the tips of your eye drop bottles clean are recommended after you have eye surgery.

When to Call the Doctor · If you develop new, severe eye pain or loss of vision after eye surgery, contact your eye surgeon the same day or go to an emergency room and ask to be seen by an eye doctor as soon as possible. Prompt diagnosis and treatment of endophthalmitis is crucial to a successful outcome.

Treatment · Endophthalmitis is treated by injecting antibiotics directly into the eye. This treatment can be performed in the office in most cases. Your doctor will try to remove a sample of vitreous for testing to find out what kind of infection is present.
In more serious cases, you may need emergency vitrectomy surgery to remove pus from the eye in addition to injection of the antibiotics.

Prognosis · With prompt treatment, patients with mild endophthalmitis after cataract surgery can recover excellent vision. Recovery can take weeks to months, and sometimes more than one antibiotic injection or more surgery is needed. In severe cases, vision may not improve, and rarely some patients may even lose the eye. The chance of visual improvement depends on the severity of the infection and on how quickly it is treated.

http://www.eyemdlink.com/Condition.asp?ConditionID=169
http://www.intelihealth.com/IH/ihtIH/WSIHW000/9339/9935.html

Epiretinal Membrane

MILA OH, M.D.

What Is It? · An epiretinal membrane (also known as macular pucker, cellophane retinopathy, or preretinal gliosis) is a thin sheet of abnormal scar tissue that grows over the retina and causes distortion of vision. Sometimes other eye conditions can cause an epiretinal membrane to form, such as inflammation, diabetes, retinal tears or detachments, previous eye surgery, or eye injury, but in many cases there is no definite cause. An epiretinal membrane can result in swelling of the macula, or central retina, which can further blur the vision.

Symptoms: What You May Experience · Your central vision will be blurred or distorted, and you may notice that straight objects appear wavy or curved.

Examination Findings: What the Doctor Looks for · After checking your vision, your eye doctor will dilate your eyes to examine your retinas for an epiretinal membrane. In some cases a special photographic test called an optical coherence tomogram, or OCT, can be done to help identify an epiretinal membrane. Another special test, called a fluorescein angiogram, may also be done to further assess the effect that the epiretinal membrane has on the macula.

What You Can Do · There is no proven way to prevent an epiretinal membrane.

When to Call the Doctor · Most epiretinal membranes are diagnosed after the patient presents to the doctor complaining of blurred central vision. Any new decrease or distortion of vision in one eye should be checked by an eye doctor.

Treatment · Most patients with mild symptoms due to epiretinal membrane do not require surgery and can have stable vision without treatment. However, if you are having problems seeing well because of the epiretinal membrane, surgery is the only proven treatment to alleviate your symptoms. Surgery involves vitrectomy (to remove the vitreous jelly) followed by membrane peeling, a technique in which the doctor uses a small tool to grab the edge of the membrane and remove it from the surface of the retina.

Prognosis: Will I See Better? · Your vision should start to slowly improve within 4 weeks of surgery and can continue to improve for up to a year after surgery. Surgery should make your vision less blurry and improve the distortion. You can usually expect to regain about half the vision that was lost because of the epiretinal membrane.

http://www.eyemdlink.com/Condition.asp?ConditionID=172
http://www.nei.nih.gov/health/pucker/

Hypertensive Retinopathy

DIANNA L. SELDOMRIDGE, M.D., MBA

What Is It? · Hypertensive retinopathy is defined as the changes that occur in the retina and retinal blood vessels as a result of hypertension (high blood pressure). Patients with hypertensive retinopathy are at risk for developing several other eye diseases, the most common of which is a retinal vein occlusion. Less commonly, one may develop a retinal arterial macroaneurysm.

Symptoms: What You May Experience · There are varying degrees of hypertensive retinopathy, the mildest of which may not noticeably affect vision. Moderate to severe hypertensive retinopathy can lead to blurry vision or vision loss in one or both eyes.

Examination Findings: What the Doctor Looks for · Your eye doctor looks for narrowing of the retinal arteries, compression of the retinal veins where arteries and veins cross, bleeding or swelling within the retina, swelling of the optic nerve, and evidence of artery blockages.

What You Can Do · The most important thing you can do is control your blood pressure with diet, exercise, and medication if your primary care doctor prescribes it.

When to Call the Doctor · Anytime you notice a change in your vision, you should make an appointment to see your doctor.

Treatment · If you develop hypertensive retinopathy, the best treatment is to control your blood pressure to prevent further damage. Currently, neither eye surgery nor glasses can improve this condition.

Prognosis: Will I See Better? · Vision loss that results from hypertensive retinopathy may be partially reversible. However, it may also become permanent, and therefore should be prevented by controlling your blood pressure.

http://www.nlm.nih.gov/medlineplus/ency/article/000999.htm
http://www.eyemdlink.com/Condition.asp?ConditionID=230

Macular Hole

BROOKS W. MCCUEN II, M.D.

What Is It? · The macula is the center of the retina and is responsible for fine vision. A macular hole is a small, full-thickness hole in the center of the retina. Macular holes usually develop in otherwise healthy patients, although they can occasionally be caused by eye injury or other eye diseases. Typically a macular hole occurs in one eye only, but about 10% of patients with a macular hole in one eye will develop a similar macular hole in their other eye.

Symptoms: What You May Experience · The retina is like the film in a camera. Seeing with a macular hole is like taking photographs with film that has a small hole in the center of the negative: the resulting photo would have a small black area in the center of the print, corresponding to the hole in the film. In a patient with a macular hole, there is a missing piece of the field of vision, shaped like a circle, when the patient looks directly at an object. That object may be missing or distorted, corresponding to the hole in the macula. Just as changing the lens on the camera would not improve the missing area in the center of the photograph if there were a hole in the film, changing the glasses for a patient with a macular hole would not eliminate the blind spot in the center of the vision.

Examination Findings: What the Doctor Looks for · If you have a macular hole you will be unable to see the small letters on the eye chart, even with the most powerful glasses correction. The eye doctor may ask you to look at a grid and say which lines may be distorted or missing. The eye doctor will dilate your pupil and examine your retina with special examining lenses, to directly see the macular hole. In some cases the eye doctor may do a fluorescein angiogram, in which a special dye is injected into one of your arm veins while photographs of your macula are taken to further study the area. A new, noninvasive method of studying macular holes is called optical coherence tomography, or OCT. This photographic test does not require any injections and is very helpful in the diagnosis and management of macular holes.

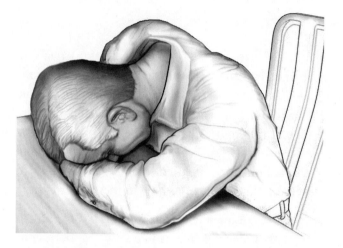

15 Some retinal surgeries require the patient to be positioned face down for several days afterward.

What You Can Do · There is no proven way to prevent the development of a macular hole. You should simply be aware of its symptoms so that if a macular hole develops, you can be examined by an eye doctor and start therapy at an early stage.

When to Call the Doctor · If you begin to notice distortion in the central vision of one of your eyes, your retina should be checked. Usually the first symptom is that straight lines begin to look crooked. Some patients who have developed a macular hole in one eye will periodically test their other eye at home with a grid given them by their eye doctor.

Treatment · The only successful treatment is surgery, called a virectomy, to close the hole. When the hole can be closed, visual function frequently stabilizes or improves. The surgeon uses tiny instruments with the help of a microscope to remove the jelly-like vitreous from the eye. Then the surgeon replaces the vitreous with a gas bubble, which if kept in contact with the macular hole will help it to close. Because the macular hole is directly in the back of the eye and because a gas bubble in the eye will always rise to the top (like a bubble in a bottle of carbonated soda), patients are asked to remain face down for a few days to several weeks after the operation. This serves to "put the bubble on the trouble" until the hole closes. The gas bubble eventually disappears completely and is replaced by the patient's own eye tissue. Rarely, silicone oil may be used instead of a gas bubble.

When the gas bubble is in the eye, it is critical not to fly in an airplane, travel to areas at high altitudes, or lie on one's back. Also, if another surgery anywhere on your body is to be performed while a gas bubble is in your eye, it is critical that the anesthesiologist know about the gas bubble so that the anesthetics used are appropriately adjusted.

Prognosis: Will I See Better? · Without surgery most patients will not experience any improvement in their vision. Modern surgery successfully closes a macular hole in about 90% of patients. When the hole is closed, most patients will experience stabilization or improvement in their central vision. Patients who have not previously had cataract surgery are highly likely to develop a cataract within months to years of macular hole surgery and will ultimately need cataract surgery for maximal improvement of their vision.

http://www.nei.nih.gov/health/macularhole/
http://www.emedicine.com/oph/topic401.htm

Retinal Artery Occlusion

SHERMAN W. REEVES, M.D., MPH

What Is It? · The blood supply for all inner layers of the retina comes from a single artery, known as the central retinal artery, which is located at the back of the eye. A blockage of the central retinal artery or any of its branches in the retina produces central or branch retinal artery occlusion.

Retinal artery occlusion can have a variety of causes. Most commonly, the artery is clogged by a small piece of debris flowing in the bloodstream. This debris often originates with the walls of diseased vessels elsewhere in the body. The debris, or embolus, could be platelets, cholesterol, or talc. Rarely, inflammation and swelling of the retinal artery itself can cause an artery occlusion.

When a retinal artery is blocked, the affected retina can no longer receive the oxygen and nourishment it needs to survive. If the blood supply is not restored within 90 minutes, the retina in this area will begin to die. As a result, the vision in that part of the eye may then be permanently lost.

Symptoms: What You May Experience · Persons who develop a retinal artery occlusion will experience the sudden, often marked onset of a decrease in their vision. The vision loss usually occurs over less than a minute and is painless.

Examination Findings: What the Doctor Looks for · Your eye doctor will check your vision, which is often poor after a retinal artery occlusion. When the retina is examined after dilation, the areas of the normally clear retina that are oxygen-starved may now appear white. A fluorescein angiogram, or photographic dye test, may be performed to help define where the occlusion has occurred.

What You Can Do · There is no proven way to reverse vision loss after a retinal artery occlusion has occurred. However, since retinal artery occlusions are often a result of atherosclerotic (cholesterol) vessel disease in other parts of the body, working with your primary medical doctor to keep your blood pressure, blood sugar, cholesterol, and weight under control can help lower your risk.

When to Call the Doctor · Any time you experience sudden loss of vision, you should see your eye doctor as soon as possible.

Treatment · Though no treatment has been shown in studies to consistently cure retinal artery occlusions, several therapies may sometimes be helpful. Your eye doctor may attempt to lower the eye pressure, which can occasionally make the blockage move further downstream in the artery and let more blood get to the retina. This may be done by massaging the eye gently, using eye drops, or sometimes draining a small amount of the aqueous humor (fluid in the anterior chamber of the eye) with a needle. After a retinal artery occlusion, your eye doctor will monitor you periodically to make sure that you do not develop further complications such as glaucoma or abnormal growth of blood vessels in the eye.

Finding the underlying cause of a retinal artery occlusion is very important. Your primary medical doctor may perform tests, such as an ultrasound of your heart or of the arteries in your neck, to look for a source of the debris that may have blocked the artery. Older patients may need blood tests to rule out inflammation of the artery that became blocked. Your primary medical doctor may also prescribe blood-thinning medications to lower your risk of future artery occlusions in the retina of the other eye or in other parts of the body.

Prognosis: Will I See Better? · Vision usually does not improve after an arterial occlusion, especially if a large part of the retina has lost its blood supply.

http://www.eyemdlink.com/Condition.asp?ConditionID=92
http://www.nlm.nih.gov/medlineplus/ency/article/001028.htm

Retinal Vein Occlusion

SHERMAN W. REEVES, M.D., MPH

What Is It? · After the retina has extracted nutrients from its blood supply, its veins transport the used blood back to the heart. Sometimes a vein in this drainage system of the retina can become clogged, causing the blood flow to back up and preventing fresh blood from entering the retina. This is called a retinal vein occlusion.

Retinal vein occlusions can have a variety of causes. Most commonly, the vein becomes blocked at a point where an artery crosses over or near the vein. Vein occlusions are often associated with high blood pressure, blood-clotting disorders, and glaucoma.

When a retinal vein is occluded and the blood flow backs up, the retina upstream from the occlusion no longer receives the proper amount of oxygen and nutrients. This can cause the retina to function poorly. If the vein occlusion is severe enough, the affected retina may die.

Retinal vein occlusions can be divided into three main types. In central retinal vein occlusion, the single main vein that drains the retina becomes blocked. In hemiretinal vein occlusion, one of the two branches of this central retinal vein becomes clogged, so blood flow from half of the retina does not drain properly. In branch retinal vein occlusion, a vein that drains a smaller portion of the retina becomes blocked, so damage primarily occurs in the area of the retina drained by that branch vein.

Symptoms: What You May Experience · Persons who develop a retinal vein occlusion may experience the sudden onset of a decrease in vision or wake up with decreased vision in one eye. The vision loss usually occurs over several minutes and is painless.

Examination Findings: What the Doctor Looks for · Those suffering from a retinal vein occlusion usually have difficulty reading the eye chart. When a dilated exam of the retina is performed, the eye doctor will often see bleeding and fluid in the retina from the backed-up veins. A fluorescein angiogram, or photographic dye test, may be performed to help define where the occlusion has occurred and define other characteristics of the vein occlusion which will help decide what to do next.

What You Can Do · Because retinal vein occlusions are often associated with other medical problems like glaucoma, high blood pressure, obesity, and cardiovascular disease, working with your eye doctor and primary medical doctor to address these problems can help lower your risk of a retinal vein occlusion in the other eye. Overall, if you develop a central retinal vein occlusion in one eye, there is 1% risk per year for the same disease to occur in the other eye. If you develop a branch retinal vein occlusion in one eye, there is a 10% risk over 3 years for the other eye to suffer a retinal vein occlusion of any type.

When to Call the Doctor · Any time you experience a sudden loss of vision, an eye doctor should see you as soon as possible. If a retinal vein occlusion has been diagnosed, any change in vision or the development of eye pain should be reported immediately to your ophthalmologist.

Treatment · Branch retinal vein occlusions can sometimes be helped by laser treatment of the macula if swelling has developed there from the blocked vein. However, no treatment has been shown in studies to consistently help eyes with central or hemiretinal vein occlusions. Several experimental surgical therapies (including injecting steroid medication into the eyeball) are now being studied. Your eye doctor will monitor you periodically after a retinal vein occlusion for possible further complications, such as glaucoma and abnormal growth of blood vessels in the eye, which may require panretinal laser photocoagulation treatment.

Prognosis: Will I See Better? · If the retinal vein occlusion is small or affects only a branch vein, vision may gradually improve over several months. However, the vision rarely returns to normal after a vein occlusion. If a central retinal vein occlusion occurs and vision is greatly decreased initially, only 20% of patients will see their vision improve; sometimes the vision even worsens over time.

http://www.geocities.com/crvo_my/
http://www.eyemdlink.com/Condition.asp?ConditionID=388

Retinal Detachment

MILA OH, M.D.

What Is It? · In a normal eye, the retina is a thin membrane that rests against the inner wall of the back of the eye, like wallpaper. The retina acts like the film of a camera, and it needs to be in its normal position to allow you to see properly. If the retina is torn, fluid can enter through this tear and accumulate underneath the retina. When this happens, the retina no longer sits on the inside wall of the eye; this is called a retinal detachment.

The macula, the central part of the retina, is important for seeing fine detail and for reading. If the macula becomes detached, permanent central vision loss can occur. For this reason, prompt treatment of retinal detachment is especially important if the macula has not yet detached.

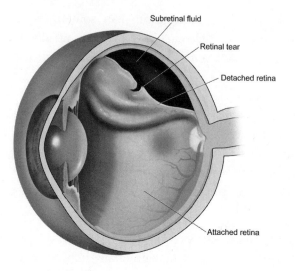

Subretinal fluid

Retinal tear

Detached retina

Attached retina

16 Retinal detachment.

People who are more at risk for retinal detachment include those who are nearsighted (myopic), have had a previous retinal detachment or tear, have had previous eye surgery or eye injury, have a family member with retinal detachment, or have new symptoms of floaters or flashes of light.

Symptoms: What You May Experience · Symptoms of a torn retina include flashes of light and floaters, which look like little moving spots in your field of vision. When the retina becomes detached, you may see a dark gray area that looks like a curtain coming over your vision from any side. This area may gradually become bigger as the retinal detachment enlarges. Retinal detachments are painless.

Examination Findings: What the Doctor Looks for · Your eye doctor will check your central vision and your side vision. Your pupils will then be dilated so that the doctor can examine your retina and look for a retinal tear or detachment.

What You Can Do · There is nothing you can do to prevent a retinal tear or detachment except avoiding eye injury.

When to Call the Doctor · If you notice new floaters or flashes of light, a dark veil coming over your vision, or decreased central vision, see your eye doctor immediately. Early treatment of a torn retina may prevent a retinal detachment, and early treatment of a retinal detachment is preferred.

Treatment · If the retina is torn but not detached, the ophthalmologist can seal the edge of the tear with laser or cryotherapy (freezing) in the office.

A retinal detachment requires surgery to put the retina back into place before sealing the torn edges. There are several ways to re-attach the retina:

Pneumatic retinopexy. Cryotherapy is performed on the retinal tear. A bubble of gas is injected into the eye and positioned to cover the treated retinal tear. This procedure is suitable for select patients and can be done in the office.

Scleral buckle. A silicone band, just like a belt, is placed around the eye to indent the wall of the eye and push the retinal tear closed. This surgery is done in the operating room.

Vitrectomy. The vitreous jelly is removed and the retina is re-attached from inside the eye by removing the fluid from underneath the retina. This surgery is also done in the operating room.

In all these procedures, a gas injection may be used to help hold the retina in place while it heals. If gas is injected into the eye, it is very important to the success of the operation that the patient maintain proper head position for up to a week, to allow the bubble to float toward the retinal tear. The patient should also avoid flying in airplanes and being at altitudes greater than 4,000 feet while the gas bubble is in the eye (up to 8 to 12 weeks). If you experience a retinal detachment that is treated with a gas injection and then need to have surgery with general anesthesia while you have gas in the eye, let the anesthesiologist know so that he or she will avoid anesthetics that might interact with the gas bubble.

Prognosis: Will I See Better? · In uncomplicated cases of retinal detachment, there is an 80–85% chance that one surgery will fix the retinal detachment. However, some patients will require more than one surgery, and some patients may not recover normal vision, especially if the macula has detached. Glasses are almost always needed to obtain the best vision possible.

http://www.nei.nih.gov/health/retinaldetach/
http://eyemdlink.com/Condition.asp?ConditionID=383

Retinitis Pigmentosa and Other Hereditary Retinal Degenerations

SCOTT BLACKMON, M.D.

What Is It? · A number of inherited eye diseases can lead to progressive damage to the retina. Retinitis pigmentosa is a group of diseases that is the most common type of retinal degeneration. With few exceptions, these disorders are passed to a child through the genes of one or both parents. Since there are many different inheritance patterns, parents may or may not have symptoms, and generations may be skipped entirely.

Symptoms: What You May Experience · The first symptom that is usually noticed is difficulty seeing in dim light. Abnormal blind spots in the vision may occur. These typically progress over time so that the peripheral vision may be lost, leading to what is often referred to as "tunnel vision." Central vision may be affected either early or late in the disease. It is rare for patients to lose all of their vision from retinitis pigmentosa.

Examination Findings: What the Doctor Looks for · The eye doctor looks for changes in the retina that are characteristic of retinitis pigmentosa. In the early stages, the eye may look relatively normal. Later, retinal pigment abnormalities commonly develop. The optic nerve may also look pale. The retinal blood vessels are narrowed, and cataracts may develop at a young age. The doctor may perform tests to confirm the diagnosis and monitor the course of the disease. An electroretinogram (ERG), for example, is a noninvasive test in which tiny sensors determine the retinal response to certain light and dark conditions. Another test is a visual field test, for side, or peripheral, vision.

What You Can Do · There is nothing proven to prevent the development of retinitis pigmentosa or other inherited retinal degenerations.

When to Call the Doctor · You should see your eye doctor if you notice changes in your central or side vision, or if you have persistent difficulty seeing in dim light. For patients with retinitis pigmentosa, it is important to have regular follow-ups with an ophthalmologist to monitor the progression of the disease, keep abreast of clinical trials and new treatment options, and learn how to adapt to decreased vision. It is important for those with retinitis pigmentosa to notify their ophthalmologist if their vision changes suddenly.

Treatment · There is currently no way to halt the progression of retinitis pigmentosa, although researchers are optimistic that an effective treatment or cure may someday be possible through genetic research. Some eye conditions that are more common in those with retinitis pigmentosa, such as cystoid macular edema and cataracts, can often be effectively treated to improve vision.

Some ophthalmologists believe that high doses of vitamin A supplements may be helpful in patients with retinitis pigmentosa, although most ophthalmologists do not believe that there is enough scientific evidence to support such a claim. High doses of vitamin A also have many potential side effects, including liver damage and birth defects.

Genetic counseling may be offered to persons with retinitis pigmentosa so that they may be well informed about having a genetically inherited disease that might be passed on to their children. Low-vision specialists can help patients function at their highest possible level despite having decreased vision. There are also support groups to help patients with decreased vision cope with their symptoms.

It is also extremely important for retinitis pigmentosa patients to have regularly scheduled visits with their primary care doctor. Occasionally, retinitis pigmentosa can be associated with other health problems, including fatal heart defects, hearing loss, kidney disorders, high cholesterol, and diabetes.

Prognosis: Will I See Better? · In general, retinitis pigmentosa and other hereditary retinal degenerations cause worsening vision over the years. However, patients with retinal degenerations may maintain some useful vision well into middle age or longer.

www.blindness.org/retinitis-pigmentosa.asp
www.emedicine.com/oph/topic704.htm

Retinoblastoma

THOMAS J. CUMMINGS, M.D.

What Is It? · Retinoblastoma is a malignant (cancerous) tumor of the primitive cells of the retina that grows in the eyeball. Although retinoblastoma is rare, it is the most common eyeball cancer in children. In the United States, there are approximately 250–500 new cases each year. Almost 90% of cases are diagnosed in children less than three years old. The younger the child when retinoblastoma is found, the greater the chance of having a family history of retinoblastoma or of having tumors in both eyes.

What Causes It? · The genetic abnormality that causes retinoblastoma has been discovered and is well described. The gene responsible for retinoblastoma is located on chromosome 13. Its normal function is to prevent tumors from growing. When the gene becomes defective, retinoblastoma can occur. Since there are several ways for the gene to become defective, the genetic cause of each patient's retinoblastoma is important for the patient's prognosis as well for family counseling (because the chance that other children in the family may get retinoblastoma is variable).

Examination Findings: What the Doctor Looks for · The classic sign of retinoblastoma is leukocoria, or a white pupil. However, the white pupil can also be seen in other eye diseases, many of which are benign (not cancerous). Other abnormal eye findings that may be associated with retinoblastoma include strabismus (crossed eyes), a red, painful eye, poor vision, a dilated pupil in only one eye, or a child's failure to grow normally. The ophthalmologist usually makes the diagnosis by examining the patient, doing radiographic studies, and asking the pathologist to examine the eye tumor if it is removed surgically.

When to Call the Doctor · A child should be examined by an ophthalmologist if he or she has a white pupil, a dilated pupil in only one eye, crossed or drifting eyes, a red, painful eye, or poor vision.

Treatment · The treatment of retinoblastoma is complex and can involve laser, freezing, or heat treatment of the tumor, plaque radiation therapy of the tumor, surgical removal of the eyeball that has the tumor, external beam radiation therapy, and chemotherapy.

Prognosis: What Are the Survival Rates? · Survival rates are excellent for children with disease confined only to the eyeball who have access to modern medical care. The risk of death from retinoblastoma is greatest if the tumor extends out of the eyeball into the orbit, brain, or bloodstream, resulting in cancer that metastasizes, or spreads, to other parts of the body. Retinoblastoma can metastasize to bones (especially in the skull), lymph nodes, and abdominal organs. Retinoblastoma patients are also at risk for developing new secondary cancers in other parts of the body as they grow older. The most common secondary cancer in retinoblastoma survivors is bone cancer, or osteogenic sarcoma.

http://www.retinoblastoma.com/frameset1.htm
http://www.acor.org/diseases/ped-onc/diseases/retino.html

Other Tumors of the Retina and Choroid

THOMAS J. CUMMINGS, M.D.

Retinal Tumors · Retinoblastoma is the most common tumor of the retina. Retinocytoma is the name of a rare tumor that can look the same as retinoblastoma on eye examination. Microscopically retinocytoma appears to be a benign (noncancerous) version of retinoblastoma, although this similarity is controversial. Other tumors of the retina are far less common and include both benign and malignant (cancerous) types. Medulloepithelioma is a rare tumor of the eye that usually occurs in children and can appear malignant under the microscope yet has a good long-term survival rate. Rare tumors called adenomas and adenocarcinomas can arise from the layer of cells between the retina and the choroid known as the retinal pigment epithelium.

Because the retina is composed of nerve tissue similar to brain tissue, tumors that more commonly occur in the brain can occasionally occur in the retina. Usually these tumors are called astrocytomas or astrocytic hamartomas and are most commonly found in patients with the disease known as tuberous sclerosis. They are typically benign and their cells resemble those of a similar brain tumor that also tends to occur in patients with tuberous sclerosis. Patients with von Hippel–Lindau disease are at risk for developing a blood vessel tumor known as retinal hemangioma or retinal hemangioblastoma, which is similar to a type of brain tumor that can also occur in von Hippel–Lindau patients. Lymphoma and leukemia can also involve the retina. Metastatic tumors to the retina, which are rare, most commonly originate with breast cancer, lung cancer, and malignant melanoma of the skin.

Choroid Tumors · The choroid is the part of the uveal tract located between the retina and the sclera where several types of tumors can occur. Metastatic cancerous tumors from other parts of the body can spread through the bloodstream to the choroid, and these tumors are the most common eyeball tumors in adults. Breast and lung cancer are the most common types of cancer to spread to the choroid.

Pigmented tumors of the choroid range from benign nevi (a nevus is like a mole on the skin) to malignant melanoma, and they are similar to skin nevi and melanoma. Malignant melanoma of the choroid usually occurs in adults and can often be found during an eye exam. Melanocytoma is a benign, pigmented tumor of the choroid that can easily be mistaken for malignant melanoma on exam; telling the difference between the two types of tumor usually requires a retina specialist who specializes in tumors of the eye. Other choroid tumors include benign lymphoid hyperplasia, which is a type of growth of the lymph tissue, and malignant lym-

.phoma, which is often associated with lymphoma in the rest of the body.

Treatment Options · The available treatments for tumors of the retina and choroid vary widely. Depending on the type, size, and location of the tumor, appropriate treatments may range from careful periodic monitoring to laser, freezing treatments, radiation, chemotherapy, or surgery. Your ophthalmologist will help you decide on the appropriate treatment for your particular situation.

http://www.eyecancer.com/
http://www.eyemdlink.com/Condition.asp?ConditionID=415

Viral Retinitis

PRITHVI MRUTHYUNJAYA, M.D.

What Is It? · A virus is an organism that lives by infecting other living cells. A virus can enter the human body through various routes — it can be inhaled in the air (influenza, or "flu," is passed in this way), ingested with food, or transmitted through contact with a living carrier of the virus. Once in the bloodstream, the virus can infect the body's cells and cause them to malfunction. However, viruses are usually attacked and controlled by the body's own immune system so that symptoms do not develop.

Viral retinitis is an extremely rare infection of the retina of one or both eyes caused by virus particles that enter the retina. Some forms of viral retinitis mainly affect patients who have systemic illnesses that weaken their own immune systems, such as Acquired Immune Deficiency Syndrome (AIDS) and cancer. Certain medications such as steroids or chemotherapy can also weaken the immune system, making a patient susceptible to viral retinitis.

There are three viruses that are commonly responsible for viral retinitis: cytomegalovirus (CMV), varicella zoster virus (HZV — the virus that causes chicken pox), and herpes simplex virus (HSV — the virus that causes cold sores). Most people are exposed to CMV and HZV as children or young adults and then become immune to them, so these viruses typically only infect the retina in patients with weakened immune systems. HSV, a common cause of cold sores, can rarely infect the retina even in otherwise healthy patients — a condition called acute retinal necrosis syndrome.

Symptoms: What You May Experience · Typically patients with viral retinitis are sensitive to light and experience floaters and possibly flashing lights in one or both eyes, along with a rapid decline in vision.

Examination Findings: What the Doctor Looks for · A dilated exam of the retina typically shows a pattern of bleeding and whitening of the normally clear retina along the blood vessels. A retinal detachment may also be present.

What You Can Do · There is nothing that can be done to prevent viral retinitis itself. Because AIDS patients are more at risk for developing viral retinitis, preventing the spread of AIDS is especially important. AIDS patients with CD4 counts of less than 50 need regular eye exams to check for early viral retinitis.

When to Call the Doctor · If you develop blurry vision and sensitivity to light, especially if you have a weakened immune system, you should call your eye doctor promptly.

Treatment · Your eye doctor will first find out if you have an underlying health condition that would predispose you to developing this type of infection and refer you to your general medical doctor for treatment. The retinal infection is usually treated for several weeks with a combination of oral, intravenous, and intraocular antiviral medications (such as ganciclovir, acyclovir, or foscarnet), depending on which virus is suspected to be the cause. In cases of CMV retinitis, an effective surgical procedure involves inserting a long-lasting pellet of ganciclovir into the vitreous to directly treat the retinal infection.

Prognosis: Will I See Better? · Although the medications used to treat viral retinitis are improving, the improvement in vision that can be achieved once the infection is controlled depends on the

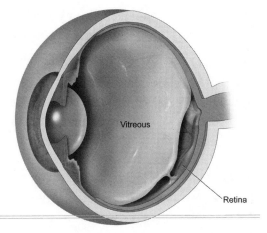

17 The vitreous gel separates from the retina in a posterior vitreous detachment.

Vitreous

Retina

severity of retinal damage caused by the virus, as well as how early the infection is diagnosed and how soon it is treated.

http://www.eyemdlink.com/EyeProcedure.asp?EyeProcedureID=57
http://www.nlm.nih.gov/medlineplus/ency/article/000665.htm

Posterior Vitreous Detachment: Flashes and Floaters

KATRINA P. WINTER, M.D. · CYNTHIA A. TOTH, M.D.

What Is It? · Posterior vitreous detachment (PVD) is the separation of the vitreous gel, which fills the eyeball behind the lens, from the inner surface of the retina. This process normally occurs as people get older and the vitreous gel begins to break down and become more liquid. Vitreous separates from the retina partially at first and can remain firmly attached to the retina in certain spots for some time before completely separating. PVD is equally common in men and women; the usual age of complete PVD is around 60 to 70. A person with high myopia (nearsightedness) is more likely to develop complete PVD at an earlier age.

Partial or complete PVD often occurs without incident and without any effect on vision. However, complete PVD rarely can distort and pull on the retina, causing a retinal tear, retinal detachment, or macular hole. Patients with a PVD but no symptoms have a low risk of developing a retinal tear or other complications.

Symptoms: What You May Experience · The most common symptoms of posterior vitreous detachment are "floaters" and "flashes." Floaters can be vitreous fibers, retinal pigment epithelial cells, or small amounts of blood that float in the vitreous. Specks of dust, cobwebs, or squiggly lines may appear to move around in your vision. Flashes, which occur especially as you move your eyes, are small bursts of light that can even be noticed in the dark. Flashes are often associated with PVD that is pulling on the retina and may be associated with the development or presence of a retinal tear or detachment.

Examination Findings: What the Doctor Looks for · Your eye doctor will dilate your eye to look for PVD and any retinal tears, retinal detachment, or other problems that it might have caused. Depending on the findings, he or she may also perform an ultrasound or optical coherence tomography (OCT) scan of your eye to help determine if the vitreous is detached from the retina.

What You Can Do · There is nothing you can do to prevent a PVD. Because retinal detachment can be hereditary, you should tell your doctor about any family history of retinal tears or detachment.

When to Call the Doctor · If you experience new floaters, an increase in the amount of floaters, flashes of light, or new distorted or blurry vision, you should contact your eye doctor.

Treatment · No treatment is required for a PVD. The patient who notices flashing lights or floaters with PVD has a higher risk of retinal tear or complications and should be scheduled for a repeat eye exam in 3–6 weeks. A retinal tear, retinal detachment, or macular hole from a PVD would require treatment.

Prognosis: Will I See Better? · A PVD by itself can cause floaters but otherwise does not affect the vision. If it causes complications such as a retinal tear or detachment or a macular hole, the vision may be affected accordingly.

http://www.medem.com/medlb/article_detaillb.cfm?article_ID=
   ZZZAZJE0G4C&sub_cat=118
http://www.eyemdlink.com/Condition.asp?ConditionID=497

Laser Treatment of Retinal Diseases

PAUL KURZ, M.D.

Laser treatments are available for many common retinal diseases. Most of these laser treatments are performed in a special laser room in the eye clinic. First, you will receive an eye drop or injection to numb the eye. Then your eye doctor or retina specialist may place a specialized contact lens on your eye as you sit with your chin in the chin rest of the laser machine. After the laser settings are adjusted, laser treatment is performed. Laser usually does not hurt.

Panretinal Laser Photocoagulation (PRP) · Some eye diseases, such as diabetic retinopathy or retinal vein occlusion, may cause the growth of abnormal new blood vessels in the eye. This is called neovascularization. Any disease that causes decreased oxygen to the retina may lead to neovascularization. Neovascularization may occur in the retina, in the back of the eye, or on the iris, in the front of the eye. Neovascularization in the back of the eye can lead to bleeding and ultimately vision loss. Iris neovascularization can lead to neovascular glaucoma with uncontrolled high eye pressure and vision loss.

Panretinal laser photocoagulation is a laser treatment that is performed if the neovascularization meets certain criteria that your eye doctor or retina specialist is trained to identify. During PRP laser is applied to the retina. Even though vision loss and complications may still occur, PRP laser decreases the chances that they will.

Rarely, patients may notice decreased vision in dim lighting, decreased side vision, or blurry central vision caused by swelling of the retina after PRP laser. Also rarely, other side effects may be noted, including a spot in the central vision, slight color vision or

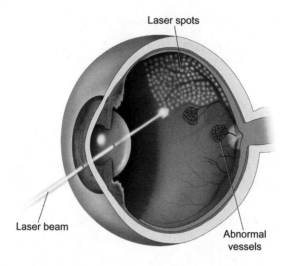

Laser spots

Laser beam

Abnormal vessels

18 Laser surgery can slow the progression of diabetic retinopathy.

contrast abnormalities, a slight decrease in the ability to focus on near objects, or a larger pupil in the treated eye. However, these side effects are generally less severe than the vision loss that may occur if neovascularization is left untreated.

During the laser treatment, you may notice a bright flash of light and possibly a slight stinging sensation each time the laser fires. If this is bothersome, an injection may be given to ease the mild discomfort. The laser treatment is usually divided into two sessions on separate days.

Focal Laser for Macular Edema · Focal laser, which may be combined with grid laser, is performed for swelling in the macula, or central retina, most is commonly caused by diabetes or branch retinal vein occlusion. Retinal swelling or thickening disrupts normal functioning, thus causing decreased vision. Focal laser is performed when the retinal swelling is causing or will likely soon cause decreased vision. The purpose of focal laser treatment is not to improve vision but to prevent vision from worsening. Rarely, vision may improve after treatment. Even more rarely, vision could worsen after treatment or the patient could notice a spot in his or her central vision. There is no pain associated with focal laser. The treated eye will usually be reevaluated several months later. Repeat treatment may be necessary.

Laser Retinopexy · Laser retinopexy involves placing laser spots around a tear in the retina to "tack down" the surrounding retina and help prevent progression to a retinal detachment. Since the laser retinopexy does not have an immediate effect, it is important to understand the symptoms of retinal detachment even after the laser treatment. If a retinal detachment does occur despite laser retinopexy, surgery in the operating room will likely be needed.

Laser Photocoagulation of Choroidal Neovascularization · Choroidal neovascularization (CNV) is a patch of abnormal blood vessels that grows under the retina in certain eye diseases such as age-related macular degeneration. If CNV occurs at or near the center of the retina, it may blur and distort the vision. Your retina specialist may first evaluate CNV with a dye test, or fluorescein angiogram. Then, if certain types of CNV occur next to but not directly in the center of the macula in the retina, laser treatment of the abnormal blood vessels may be indicated.

Immediately after this treatment, you will most likely note a permanent blind spot in your vision where the treatment was applied. The rationale for performing this treatment is to destroy the CNV before it involves the very center of your vision, which could decrease vision further and make treatment with laser more debilitating.

Photodynamic Therapy for Choroidal Neovascularization · For certain types of CNV affecting the center of the macula in the retina, photodynamic therapy (PDT) may be indicated. This treatment involves a machine similar to a laser that uses special light rays. The first step is to administer a dye (verteporfin) through a vein in the arm over 10 minutes; 5 minutes after the dye is finished infusing, the laser is applied for 83 seconds to the CNV where the dye has collected. The special dye and light prevent damage to the normal surrounding retina. It may require 5 or more treatments over approximately 24 months to treat the CNV completely.

One side effect that 2% of patients experience is lower back pain upon infusion of the dye. The cause of the back pain is not known. In addition, after photodynamic therapy, the patient must stay out of direct sunlight or bright lights for 5 days. The goal of this treatment is to stabilize vision.

Other Laser Treatments · Other eye diseases, such as retinal artery macroaneurysm or retinal capillary hemangioma, can also be treated with laser if the center of the macula in the retina and thus vision are affected.

www.visudyne.com
http://www.nei.nih.gov/health/diabetic/retinopathy.asp

Retinal Surgery

VINCENT A. DERAMO, M.D.

Eye surgery has made great advances in recent years. Today there are numerous eye conditions and diseases that can benefit from surgery. Many eye surgeries, such as cataract surgery and corneal transplantation, involve the front portion of the eye. Retinal surgery is performed on the back portion of the eye. Only your eye doctor can determine whether an eye would benefit from retinal surgery. In general, there are two basic types of retinal surgery: vitrectomy and scleral buckling.

Vitrectomy · The vitreous cavity occupies over 80% of the eye's volume and contains a gel-like material. Surgical removal of the vitreous gel from this cavity is called vitrectomy. The vitreous is not needed to see well and can safely be removed if necessary. Because the vitreous gel is involved in many retinal disorders, such as diabetic retinopathy, retinal detachment, macular hole, epiretinal membrane, hemorrhage, retained lens material, dislocated lens implant, infection, inflammation, severe eye injury, and intraocular foreign bodies, among others, vitrectomy may benefit some eyes with these conditions.

As with any medical procedure, there are risks associated with vitrectomy which your surgeon will review with you. The surgery

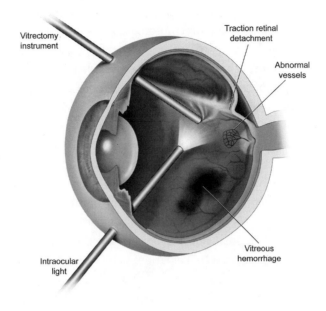

Vitrectomy instrument

Traction retinal detachment

Abnormal vessels

Intraocular light

Vitreous hemorrhage

19 Instruments placed in eyeball for vitrectomy surgery.

is performed in an operating room with either local or general anesthesia. Under local anesthesia, the patient is awake but sedated, and a numbing medicine is placed around the operated eye. Most patients find this comfortable without any significant pain during the procedure. In other cases, especially in young patients, general anesthesia is used so that the patient sleeps throughout the procedure.

Vitrectomy is performed using a microscope, often with the aid of an assistant. The eye is dilated and the surgeon is able to see the retina through the enlarged pupil.

After the eye is cleaned with a sterilizing soap solution, three very small incisions are made in the sclera, or white, outer layer of the eyeball. An infusion line is placed through one of these incisions to allow saline to flow into the eye and replace the vitreous gel during surgery. Very small instruments, such as a vitreous cutter, which is a specialized instrument that removes the vitreous gel without harming the retina, are placed through the other two incisions to allow the surgeon to work on the eye. Other frequently used instruments are an illuminating light source, a laser probe, and specialized micro-scissors. Other retinal procedures, such as laser treatment, membrane peeling (removal of scar tissue), removal of cataract or retained lens material, and administration of certain drugs into the vitreous cavity, can be done at the same time as vitrectomy.

At the end of vitrectomy, it is sometimes necessary to place an air or gas bubble in the vitreous cavity. This bubble helps to hold the retina in place while it heals. Depending on the type of gas chosen by the surgeon, the bubble will last from a few days to many weeks before it dissolves completely on its own. While the bubble is present, the surgeon may ask the patient to hold his or her head in a certain position, such as face down or right or left side down. It is very important that a patient with a bubble avoid flying in an airplane or traveling to very high altitudes, since the bubble can expand and injure the eye. Also, a patient with a bubble needs to alert other doctors if he or she requires surgery elsewhere on the body.

In other cases, silicone oil is used to fill the vitreous cavity. Silicone oil does not dissolve or disappear on its own, so it may need to be removed in a subsequent operation.

After vitrectomy the eye may feel "scratchy" or irritated for a few days. The surgeon will prescribe eye drops for use after surgery. Typically the eye is reexamined the day after surgery and then periodically. Complete healing can take from weeks to several months.

Scleral Buckling · In scleral buckling, a permanent band called a buckle is placed around the eyeball, like a belt, to support the retina in proper position. Buckles have been safely used for many years and are well tolerated by the eye. Unlike vitrectomy, which is used to treat several retinal disorders, scleral buckling is mainly used to repair retinal detachment. As in vitrectomy, there are risks associated with surgery that your surgeon will discuss with you. The surgery is performed in an operating room, with either local or general anesthesia.

During surgery, the eye is first cleaned with a sterilizing soap solution. Your surgeon examines the retina during surgery to determine where the retinal detachment and any retinal tears that may have caused it are located. These retinal tears may be treated with cryotherapy, which is a freezing treatment that helps the retina to remain in proper position. Then the scleral buckle is placed around the eyeball. The buckle itself is a permanent piece of flexible material, often solid silicone rubber or silicone sponge. The buckle is stitched into place around the eyeball, supporting the retina and repairing the detachment. The buckle is not visible after surgery, as it is placed far back on the eye, behind the eyelids. Fluid under the detached retina may also be drained during surgery to help the retina reattach to the eye wall.

Sometimes, as in vitrectomy, an air or gas bubble is used in scleral buckling, and the surgeon may ask the patient to hold his or her head in a certain position, such as face down or right or left side down. Also as in vitrectomy, the eye may feel irritated or "scratchy" for a few days after surgery. The patient is started on eye drops and the eye is typically reexamined the day after surgery, then periodically.

If you are undergoing retinal surgery, you will likely have further questions which should be discussed with your surgeon. In many cases, retinal surgery is extremely valuable in restoring vision lost because of severe retinal diseases that were untreatable in the not-so-distant past.

http://www.eyemdlink.com/EyeProcedure.asp?EyeProcedureID=58
http://www.eyemdlink.com/EyeProcedure.asp?EyeProcedureID=52

10 · Inflammation of the Eyeball

Uveitis

PRITHVI MRUTHYUNJAYA, M.D.

What Is It? · Uveitis means inflammation of the uveal tract, which is the pigmented portion of the eyeball composed of the choroid, ciliary body, and iris. These structures all have an abundant blood supply, which may make them susceptible to inflammation and infections from other parts of the body. Our individual immune systems play an important role in determining the development and severity of the inflammation, so episodes of uveitis will be different in each patient.

The most common classification of uveitis is based on the structures that are inflamed. Anterior uveitis (also called iritis or iridocyclitis) is inflammation in the front of the eye, in the anterior chamber and iris; intermediate uveitis (also called pars planitis) is inflammation in the front and middle part of the eye, in the anterior chamber, iris, and part of the vitreous cavity; posterior uveitis involves the back part of the eye in the retina and vitreous; and panuveitis involves all structures, from the front to the back of the eyeball.

Uveitis may be caused or made worse by eye injury or various systemic illnesses, including infections and autoimmune diseases (when the body's immune system begins to attack its own uveal tract). In the majority of cases, a specific cause cannot be identified despite a careful medical examination and laboratory testing. Your doctor will still try to determine the exact reason why the uveitis occurred so that he or she will be able to treat the underlying cause as well as the inflammation itself.

Symptoms: What You May Experience · In general, patients experience eye pain, redness, light sensitivity, and blurry vision. In posterior uveitis and panuveitis there is a greater chance of having decreased vision, because the choroid toward the back of the eye is affected.

Examination Findings: What the Doctor Looks for · Your eye doctor will ask about your medical history. Because all parts of the eye can be affected, a complete dilated eye exam is performed to assess the degree of inflammation in different parts of the eye. Your eye doctor will look specifically for inflammatory cells floating in your eyeball. The eye pressure is measured, since uveitis can sometimes cause glaucoma. Additional testing, including fluorescein angiography and ultrasound, may be performed. In some cases your doctor may order laboratory tests to help identify the cause of the uveitis. An evaluation by your primary medical doctor may also be required. In very severe cases, a sample of eye fluid may be removed with vitrectomy surgery and tested to determine the exact cause of the inflammation.

What You Can Do · Avoiding eye injury helps to prevent uveitis. If you have an underlying systemic autoimmune disease, controlling it with the help of your medical doctor may help to prevent uveitis in the future.

When to Call the Doctor · If you develop eye pain and redness, blurry vision, or new light sensitivity, you should contact your eye doctor.

Treatment · Typically your eye doctor will begin treatment with frequent steroid eye drops (up to once every hour), which will be gradually used less often over weeks to months. Sometimes severe inflammation (usually in posterior uveitis or panuveitis) may require oral steroids or steroid injections around the eyeball. Your doctor will monitor you for any harmful eye and systemic side effects that can be caused by all forms of steroid medications (such as cataract and glaucoma in the eye). In the most severe cases of uveitis, oral or injected immunosuppressive medicines are prescribed, typically with the assistance of your primary medical doctor or rheumatologist. Your doctor will treat any other infections or illnesses that he or she believes may be related to your uveitis.

Prognosis: Will I See Better? · Uveitis can be a long-standing, recurrent inflammatory condition. The severity and extent of the inflammation will determine the extent of improvement. Prompt diagnosis and treatment with steroids will often restore vision to excellent levels. If you have uveitis, it is important to follow your doctor's instructions about your prescribed medications and to inform him or her immediately of any changes in your vision.

http://www.eyemdlink.com/Condition.asp?ConditionID=510
http://www.nlm.nih.gov/medlineplus/ency/article/001005.htm

Episcleritis

PRITHVI MRUTHYUNJAYA, M.D.

What Is It? · The episclera is the connective tissue layer underneath the clear conjunctiva that overlies the white sclera. The small fibers in the episclera can become inflamed, a condition termed episcleritis. The majority of cases are not caused by any systemic disease or eye infection.

Symptoms: What You May Experience · Episcleritis often causes eye irritation, tearing, and itching. It rarely causes severe eye pain, discharge, or decreased vision. Usually a small area of the white part of the eyeball will appear red.

Examination Findings: What the Doctor Looks for · Using the slit lamp, your eye doctor can identify any episcleral inflammation while ruling out infection, glaucoma, or inflammation inside the eyeball (uveitis). He or she may confirm the diagnosis of episcleritis by using a dilating eye drop.

What You Can Do · There is no way to prevent the development of episcleritis.

When to Call the Doctor · If you notice eye redness that is associated with discharge, eye pain, or decreased vision, call your eye doctor promptly. Persistent eye redness by itself may be examined more routinely.

Treatment · Episcleritis usually resolves within a week even without treatment. For comfort, artificial tears may be used, but medicated eye drops designed to reduce eye redness should be avoided, as they can worsen the condition in the long run. In severe cases, a steroid eye drop may be prescribed for a short time to control the inflammation. Oral anti-inflammatory medicines such as ibuprofen may also be prescribed in recurrent cases.

Prognosis: Will I See Better? · Although episcleritis usually resolves quickly without permanent consequences, some patients experience repeated episodes. It is important to inform your eye doctor if your symptoms return.

http://www.emedicine.com/oph/topic641.htm
http://www.eyemdlink.com/Condition.asp?ConditionID=173

Scleritis

PRITHVI MRUTHYUNJAYA, M.D.

What Is It? · Scleritis is inflammation of the sclera, the white, outer covering of the eyeball. This rare condition can affect either the front (anterior scleritis) or back (posterior scleritis) of the eye. Scleritis differs from other causes of a red eye because of its possible association with infections as well as systemic diseases such as rheumatoid arthritis and systemic lupus erythematosis.

Symptoms: What You May Experience · Scleritis often causes severe eye pain, decreased vision, and floaters. In anterior scleritis, the normally white part of the eyeball is typically red, either in a small area or all over. In posterior scleritis, vision may be severely decreased while the front of the eye can show little or no redness.

Examination Findings: What the Doctor Looks for · Anterior scleritis is diagnosed by examination with a slit lamp. The pattern of redness helps to classify the scleritis, while thinning of the sclera or cornea indicates more severe disease. Your eye doctor may dilate your pupils to look for posterior scleritis or other inflammation in the back of the eye. In posterior scleritis, ultrasound testing, fluorescein angiography (a photographic dye test), or a computed tomography (CT) scan can sometimes aid in making the diagnosis. Your eye doctor may order blood tests to determine if the scleritis is related to underlying systemic inflammation or infection and may recommend an evaluation by your primary medical doctor.

What You Can Do · There is no proven way to avoid the development of scleritis.

When to Call the Doctor · If you notice eye redness that is associated with discharge, eye pain, or decreased vision, call your eye doctor promptly. He or she may refer you to an eye M.D. who specializes in uveitis.

Treatment · Oral nonsteroidal anti-inflammatory drugs (NSAIDS), such as indomethacin and ibuprofen, are the first line of treatment in scleritis. Steroid eye drops may be prescribed in some cases as well. In more severe cases, oral steroids and other systemic immunosuppressive medicines (such as cyclosporine and methotrexate) may be used. Complications from scleritis such as thinning of the eye wall or perforation may require eye surgery.

Prognosis: Will I See Better? · In cases of mild to moderate scleritis, you can maintain or recover excellent vision. In more severe cases, the type of scleritis, how long the inflammation lasts, and complications from either disease or treatment will determine the extent of improvement. Follow-up visits with your primary medical doctor are essential for any associated systemic illness.

http://eyemdlink.com/Condition.asp?ConditionID=400
http://www.intelihealth.com/IH/ihtIH/WSIHW000/9339/9957.html

11 · The Optic Nerve

Glaucoma

CLAUDIA S. COHEN, M.D.

What Is It? · Glaucoma is a leading cause of blindness in the United States. It is progressive, and quite often a person with glaucoma will be completely unaware of the disease until it is quite advanced. Fortunately, if glaucoma is detected early enough, it can be treated.

Glaucoma is four to six times more common in black patients, but people of all ethnic backgrounds are at risk. Family history is a significant risk factor. It is important to tell your ophthalmologist if anyone in your family has had glaucoma. In the past, glaucoma has been associated with high eye pressure. While there are many patients who do have glaucoma and high eye pressure, it is possible to have normal eye pressure and still have glaucoma.

Symptoms: What You May Experience · Primary open-angle glaucoma, the most common type, is typically symptom-free at first, and therefore the patient may not realize that the disease is present until it has already damaged the vision substantially. This is because glaucoma progresses gradually, and typically affects peripheral vision before it affects central vision. Once a patient starts to lose any vision, about 30–50% of the optic nerve has already been permanently damaged. There is no treatment that can restore vision once it is lost because of glaucoma.

Some types of glaucoma may be associated with eye pain. Usually the pain is rather significant, and the patient will typically seek medical care the same day.

Examination Findings: What the Doctor Looks for · An ophthalmologist is trained to look for signs of glaucoma before symptoms appear. An important part of the eye exam is measuring the eye

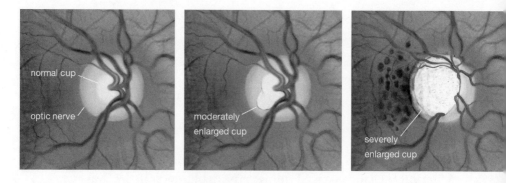

20 Left: normal optic nerve. Center: optic nerve with moderate glaucoma.
Right: optic nerve with severe glaucoma.

pressure. The normal range for eye pressure is 10–22 mm Hg. However, some people typically have eye pressures above the normal range, while other people have normal eye pressures but may still be at risk for glaucoma.

If you do have higher eye pressure than expected, your ophthalmologist may measure the thickness of your cornea. This measurement is called pachymetry. Recent studies have found that the thickness of the cornea varies among individuals. Corneal thickness may have an effect on the measurement of eye pressure.

The dilated eye exam is the next step that the ophthalmologist will use to assess your optic nerve. You should have an experienced doctor perform this part of the eye examination, as there may be subtle clues that can easily be missed. If your ophthalmologist suspects that you have glaucoma, often photographs of your optic nerves will be taken so that there will be a standard for comparison during future exams.

If your eye doctor suspects that you have glaucoma based on the appearance of your optic nerve, your eye pressures, or both, you will be asked to perform a computerized visual field test. This is a test to see if you are missing part of your peripheral vision, or visual field. In this test, you sit in a dimly lit room and look into a white bowl. You will see flashing lights in your peripheral vision and will be asked to press a button each time you see the light.

The test can be quite challenging and tiring, so you may be asked to come back at another time to repeat it.

What You Can Do · Even if you do not have known glaucoma, the most important thing you can do is to visit your ophthalmologist at least once every 1–2 years. Because glaucoma is a slowly progressive disease, small changes may be apparent from year to year. It is also helpful if you know your family history. There is a genetic component to glaucoma, so if you have a family member with it, you may be more likely to have it yourself.

If you have known glaucoma, you should use your eye drops as prescribed and follow up with your eye doctor regularly.

When to Call the Doctor · Glaucoma is a disease that can take many years to develop. Because there are virtually no symptoms, it is unlikely to require an emergency visit to your ophthalmologist. Should you have reason to think you may have glaucoma, you need to call your ophthalmologist and make an appointment for a routine eye examination. If you develop sudden, intense eye pain that lasts longer than several seconds, you should see your eye doctor right away, because certain types of glaucoma can present in this way.

Treatment · Once it has been determined that you have glaucoma, you will likely be started on an eye drop to lower your eye pressure. There are many types of drops available, and your doctor will choose the one that best suits you. Typically you will be asked to return several weeks later to see how well the medicine is working. If it is working well, you are usually seen every few months. If your eye pressure is still too high, another type of eye drop may be added. There are also treatments involving laser and other types of surgery.

Prognosis: Will I See Better? · Once glaucoma has done its damage to the optic nerve, these cells cannot regenerate, or come back. A patient's prognosis depends on the stage at which the disease was diagnosed, and prognosis varies greatly among patients. At this time, glaucoma treatment is designed to prevent vision loss from worsening rather than to regain the vision that has been already lost.

www.nei.nih.gov/health/glaucoma/glaucoma-facts.asp
www.iga.org.uk/servlet/dycon/iga/iga/live/en/uk/home

Laser Treatment of Glaucoma

CLAUDIA S. COHEN, M.D.

What Is It? · One method of surgically treating glaucoma is to use a laser. There are several types of laser treatment available. Laser surgery is often indicated if pressure-lowering eye drops are not able to keep the eye pressure in a safe range. Sometimes patients are not able to tolerate eye drops, or damage to the optic nerve worsens despite maximal use of medications. When this occurs, alternative treatments must be used. The two most common glaucoma laser treatments are laser trabeculoplasty and laser peripheral iridectomy.

Laser trabeculoplasty is used in patients with primary openangle glaucoma, the most common form of glaucoma. Laser trabeculoplasty may also be beneficial in patients with several subtypes of glaucoma, including pseudoexfoliation and pigmentary glaucoma. The laser is used to improve the natural drainage of aqueous fluid from the eye, thus lowering the eye pressure.

Patients who present with acute angle closure glaucoma, a rarer type of glaucoma often associated with eye pain and decreased vision, will usually require a tiny hole to be made in the iris to relieve the eye pressure. This hole is called a peripheral iridectomy and is usually performed with a laser as well.

What You May Experience during the Procedure · Laser surgery is done in the clinic, and usually the only required anesthesia is a numbing eye drop. Your ophthalmologist will hold a special contact lens on your eye to help aim the laser beam. Although you may feel the contact lens against your eyelids, there is usually no pain associated with the laser treatment. It is important that you hold very still while the ophthalmologist is performing the laser surgery. The entire procedure typically takes only a few minutes, and most patients are pleasantly surprised that it is over so quickly. Your eye doctor may ask you to use a steroid eye drop for several days after the laser treatment to help prevent inflammation.

Possible Complications · Although complications are rare, it is important to recognize that they can occur. The most common complication after laser surgery is high eye pressure. Your ophthalmologist may give you a pressure-lowering eye drop before the laser to help avoid this problem. In addition, you may be asked to stay in the clinic for 30–60 minutes after your procedure to have your eye pressure measured. About 20% of patients will have increased eye pressure immediately after the treatment, but this generally resolves quickly with eye drops. Inflammation in the eye can also occur after laser treatment, but this usually resolves with steroid eye drops.

Prognosis: Will I See Better? · As with most glaucoma treatments, patients typically do not notice an improvement in their vision. The goal of glaucoma therapy is to prevent further loss of vision. Typically your ophthalmologist waits 4–6 weeks after the initial laser treatment to assess how well it has worked and whether more laser treatment is needed. Not all glaucoma patients respond equally well to laser treatment, but most patients who undergo laser trabeculoplasty will see a decrease in their eye pressure for approximately 6–12 months after the treatment. About half the patients who responded well initially to laser trabeculoplasty will continue to have good effects from the laser over the next 3–5 years.

http://www.medem.com/MedLB/article_detaillb.cfm?article_ID=
ZZZ55FH7HEC&sub_cat=38

http://www.iga.org.uk/servlet/dycon/iga/iga/live/en/uk/
AboutGlaucoma_TreatingGlaucoma_questions

Glaucoma Surgery

CLAUDIA S. COHEN, M.D.

What Is It? · One method of treating glaucoma is with incisional, rather than laser, surgery. The most common operation of this type is called a trabeculectomy. This option is usually chosen when other treatment options such as pressure-lowering eye drops or a laser procedure (for certain patients) have not achieved the ideal degree of pressure lowering. The goal of trabeculectomy is to create a new passage that will allow the aqueous fluid to drain from the anterior chamber of the eye, thus decreasing eye pressure. Certain medicines may be used at the time of surgery to make the trabeculectomy more effective by slowing down the body's natural healing response, which otherwise might scar down the drainage passage too quickly.

Other surgical options for treating glaucoma include placing tube shunts in the eye to create new drainage pathways for the aqueous fluid.

What You May Experience during the Procedure · Incisional surgery is performed in an operating room. Like many eye surgeries, glaucoma operations are typically outpatient procedures performed under local anesthesia with intravenous sedation. This means that you will be breathing on your own but you will be very relaxed and should not feel any pain during the procedure. If you experience any discomfort, you should immediately notify your surgeon so that you can receive more numbing medication or anesthetics.

Possible Complications · The challenge in performing glaucoma surgery is that a number of complications may occur. During the surgery itself the risks are relatively low but do include bleeding, infection, and in extremely rare cases loss of the eye itself. If complications do arise, they typically occur in the days to weeks following the surgery and are generally treatable.

Because a new drainage passage has been created in a trabeculectomy, aqueous fluid can sometimes overfilter or leak and cause low eye pressure, or hypotony. There are a number of interventions your ophthalmologist may use to help correct this problem. Sometimes you may require an extra stitch, a change in your eye drops, or a bandage contact lens for days or weeks after the surgery. Leaks can occur even years after the original trabeculectomy procedure.

In other situations, the pressure may remain too high as your body attempts to scar down the new drainage passage during the natural healing process. You may be asked to perform specialized massage to the eye periodically to help lower the pressure. Often your ophthalmologist will cut one or more stitches with a laser, to help open the drainage passage and let more aqueous fluid drain out. This procedure is usually done in the clinic.

As with any type of eye surgery, the potential for infection always exists. This risk may remain present even years after a trabeculectomy is performed. It is important to immediately notify your ophthalmologist if you notice any vision loss, increasing eye pain, or increasing eye redness or discharge, as these may signify a serious infection.

Prognosis: Will I See Better? · As with any glaucoma treatment, the goal is to prevent further visual loss. Soon after glaucoma surgery, the vision may be a bit worse than before the surgery, as the eye takes several weeks to recover. The vision usually will not improve beyond the baseline, as the glaucoma damage that has already been done to the optic nerve cannot be reversed. The goal of glaucoma surgery is to save the vision that remains.

http://www.nei.nih.gov/health/glaucoma/glaucoma_facts.asp
http://www.iga.org.uk/servlet/dycon/iga/iga/live/en/uk/
  AboutGlaucoma_TreatingGlaucoma_questions

Optic Neuritis

DAVID A. CHESNUTT, M.D.

What Is It? · Optic neuritis is a specific type of optic neuropathy in which the optic nerve becomes inflamed. Several types of inflammation may involve the optic nerve. Some of these types of inflammation may affect other parts of the body, including the central nervous system (the brain, the spinal cord, and their nerves). Optic neuritis occurs most commonly in young adult females.

One disease sometimes associated with optic neuritis is multiple sclerosis. In multiple sclerosis, there are repeated bouts of inflammation in various parts of the central nervous system, including the optic nerve.

Symptoms: What You May Experience · Most patients with optic neuritis will have eye pain. The pain is often severe and worsens when the patient moves or touches the eye. The pain is usually accompanied by blurred vision and difficulty in distinguishing colors.

Examination Findings: What the Doctor Looks for · Your eye doctor will perform specific tests to evaluate the optic nerve. These tests may include vision and color vision testing, evaluation of your side vision, and direct examination of the optic nerve itself after dilating your pupils. Because optic neuritis may be part of a more widespread inflammatory process, your doctor may order blood tests or magnetic resonance imaging (MRI) scans of your brain and orbits.

What You Can Do · There is no proven way to prevent optic neuritis. If you have or suspect you may have optic neuritis, tell your eye doctor about any other symptoms that you may be experiencing in other parts of your body, in case these symptoms signify inflammation elsewhere.

When to Call the Doctor · If you experience eye pain, blurred vision, or difficulty distinguishing colors, call your eye doctor. Prompt medical attention often helps to preserve vision.

Treatment · Since optic neuritis involves inflammation of the optic nerve, you may receive anti-inflammatory medications such as steroids. These medications are often given intravenously at first, either at home or in the hospital, sometimes followed by oral steroids. Your eye doctor may also refer you to a neurologist, especially in cases where multiple sclerosis is involved or suspected.

Prognosis: Will I See Better? · Most patients who experience optic neuritis do recover vision. The vision may return completely to normal or may improve partially. A small number of patients with optic neuritis may experience permanent visual loss. Optic neuritis can recur in 28% of cases.

www.djo.harvard.edu/OA/ON/ON.html
www.albany.net/~tjc/hla_on_ms.html www.nationalmssociety.org

Optic Neuropathy

DAVID A. CHESNUTT, M.D.

What Is It? · Optic neuropathy is defined as abnormal function of the optic nerve, which serves as the connector between the eye and brain. The optic nerve transmits visual information that has been gathered by the eye to the brain, which processes this information and forms the images that we see. There are many causes of optic neuropathy, including blood flow problems, inflammation, infection, injury, inherited diseases, glaucoma, and tumors compressing the optic nerve.

Symptoms: What You May Experience · If you have an optic neuropathy, your vision may be blurred, colors may appear faded, and there may be blind spots in your field of vision. These changes can occur suddenly or gradually, and eye pain is occasionally present.

Examination Findings: What the Doctor Looks for · Your eye doctor will check your level of vision, your side vision, and your pupils, which will then be dilated so that he or she can examine your optic nerves directly. If there is any evidence of problems with optic nerve function, your eye doctor may perform more specialized testing, including color vision testing, more extensive side vision examination, blood tests, or special x-rays (CT or MRI scans) of your brain and orbits.

What You Can Do · Because there are so many possible causes of optic neuropathy, only some causes can be prevented. Optic neuropathy caused by injury can sometimes be avoided by wearing eye protection. Controlling your general health, such as your cholesterol level, blood pressure, and blood sugar if you are diabetic, can help to prevent optic neuropathy caused by blood flow problems. Being alert to the symptoms of optic neuropathy can lead to earlier treatment, which may help to preserve vision.

When to Call the Doctor · If you notice decreased central or side vision, difficulty distinguishing colors, or eye pain, call your eye doctor. Early diagnosis and treatment can often prevent problems from progressing.

Treatment · Treatment of optic neuropathy depends on the specific cause. Optic neuropathy caused by blood flow problems may be treated with blood thinning medications, such as aspirin, to protect the other eye. Optic neuropathy caused by inflammation or injury may be treated with anti-inflammatory or steroid medications. Infections that cause optic neuropathy may require antibiotics, and glaucoma may respond to medications that lower the eye pressure. If a tumor compresses the optic nerve and causes an optic neuropathy, surgery may be indicated to remove the tumor.

Prognosis: Will I See Better? · Depending on the cause, certain optic neuropathies may be successfully treated, while other optic neuropathies are more difficult or even impossible to treat once optic nerve damage has occurred. In many cases, however, treatment may at least prevent the progression of vision loss, so early diagnosis is extremely important.

www.ifond.org www.lowvision.org/ischemic_optic_neuropathy.htm

Papilledema

DAVID A. CHESNUTT, M.D.
What Is It? · Papilledema is a condition in which the optic nerves, which are the connectors between the eyes and the brain, become swollen as a result of elevated pressure from the fluid that normally surrounds the brain and spinal cord. The same fluid, called cerebrospinal fluid (CSF), also surrounds both optic nerves.

Papilledema has a variety of causes. Elevated cerebrospinal fluid pressure can be a side effect of certain medicines, such as tetracycline and some hormonal medications. Pseudotumor cerebri is a disease in which the cerebrospinal fluid pressure is elevated without a known cause; it most commonly occurs in young, overweight women. In rare cases, a mass or tumor in the brain leads to the elevated pressure.

Symptoms: What You May Experience · You may experience brief episodes of visual blackout or dimming that last only for a few seconds and affect one or both eyes. Even though the vision often returns, these episodes may lead to permanent loss of vision if not treated appropriately. You may also notice double vision if the elevated fluid pressure damages the nerves that control eye movements. Severe headaches, nausea, and vomiting may accompany papilledema.

Examination Findings: What the Doctor Looks for · In the early stages papilledema often does not cause any symptoms. Your eye doctor may see swelling of your optic nerves after dilating your pupils as part of the regular complete eye exam. If both optic nerves are swollen, a special x-ray (CT or MRI) is usually performed to determine the cause of the increased pressure around the optic nerves. A spinal tap may then be performed, to analyze the cerebrospinal fluid and measure its pressure.

What You Can Do · Pseudotumor cerebri is one preventable cause of papilledema. Avoiding obesity helps prevent and treat most cases of pseudotumor cerebri.

When to Call the Doctor · If you notice episodes of vision loss, double vision, severe headaches, or nausea and vomiting, seek medical attention promptly. Early recognition of papilledema is important to preserve vision in the long run.

Treatment · The treatment of papilledema depends on the cause. If a certain medicine is thought to be causing the elevated pressure, then that medicine may need to be discontinued. If pseudotumor cerebri is the cause, weight loss and a medication called acetazolamide, or Diamox, may be prescribed to help reduce the fluid pressure. In severe cases of pseudotumor cerebri, surgery to relieve the pressure on the optic nerves may be necessary. This surgery may involve either decompression of the optic nerve sheath (a procedure in which the tissue surrounding the optic nerve is slit to relieve pressure on the nerve) or a special shunt to drain fluid from around the brain or spinal cord. Papilledema caused by a brain tumor requires treatment of the tumor.

Prognosis: Will I See Better? · In many cases papilledema can be successfully treated to maintain good vision or help restore lost vision to some extent. However, it is critical to diagnose and treat papilledema early, before the optic nerves are irreversibly damaged.

http://www.eyemdlink.com/Condition.asp?ConditionID=340
www.intelihealth.com/IH/ihtIH/WSIHW000/9339/10463.html

12 · The Eye Muscles

Strabismus (Crossed Eyes)

LAURA ENYEDI, M.D.

What Is It? · Strabismus is a condition in which both eyes are not pointed in the same direction. One or both eyes may cross in toward the nose (esotropia), out toward the ear (exotropia), upward (hypertropia), or downward (hypotropia). The misalignment may be constant or may come and go, varying from day to day or even over the course of a day.

Strabismus can occur at any age and is common, affecting 2–5% of the population. Strabismus is often seen in children and may be present at birth or develop in the first few years of life. The cause of most childhood strabismus is unknown.

Eye movements are normally controlled by six muscles that are attached to each eyeball. For the eyes to focus together, the brain must coordinate the actions of all twelve muscles so that they work perfectly together and point both eyeballs in the same direction. Children with disorders that affect the brain such as cerebral palsy, Down syndrome, hydrocephalus, or brain tumors are more likely to develop strabismus than other children. There is also an increased risk of strabismus in children who have a family history of strabismus, who are born prematurely, or who have other eye disorders such as cataract.

Symptoms: What You May Experience · Normal alignment of the eyes is critical for normal visual development. Strabismus in children is often associated with poor visual development (amblyopia), which may be permanent. Strabismus also interferes with the ability to use the eyes together and can affect depth perception. Young children do not usually notice any problems with their vision and will often have no symptoms other than a tendency for

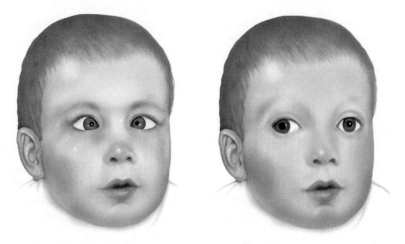

21 Left: the eyes cross in toward the nose in esotropia.
Right: the eyes drift out toward the ears in exotropia.

the eyes not to move together. Sometimes a child will squint one eye in bright sunlight or tilt his or her head because of strabismus. In older children and adults, strabismus often causes double vision (diplopia).

Examination Findings: What the Doctor Looks for · Anyone with strabismus needs a full eye exam. Even infants can be examined, using specialized techniques. The eye doctor will determine how the eyes are working together, the amount of the misalignment, the vision in each eye, and the refraction (need for glasses). The eyes will be dilated and fully examined for other serious diseases such as cataracts or eye tumors that can cause strabismus in children.

What You Can Do · Strabismus is not a preventable condition. Take your child for an eye exam at least once by the age of 6.

When to Call the Doctor · It is critical that childhood strabismus be diagnosed and treated early. If you suspect that your child has strabismus, you should immediately take him or her to an ophthalmologist for a full examination. Very young infants' eyes often do not focus together and may occasionally wander, but after the age of 3 months your child's eyes should focus together and be aligned. If the eyes are not straight by this age, your child should be examined by an ophthalmologist. An adult who develops strabismus or double vision also needs prompt examination by an ophthalmologist to diagnose possible serious diseases such as brain tumor or stroke that can cause eye misalignments.

Treatment · Strabismus is not outgrown and usually does not improve without treatment. In young children, early treatment is critical for proper vision development. Various treatments may be used alone or in combination, depending on the type and cause of the strabismus. Strabismus treatment is often combined with amblyopia treatment. Glasses are commonly prescribed for farsighted children, and double vision in adults can sometimes be relieved by using prisms in the glasses. Occasionally medications in the form of eye drops or injections into the eye muscles are used to treat strabismus. Surgery to realign the eye muscles is frequently necessary for both children and adults. Often both eyes require eye muscle surgery, and more than one surgery may be necessary to align the eyes.

Prognosis: Will I See Better? · With proper prompt treatment, strabismus can be corrected or alleviated in many cases.

www.aapos.org www.preventblindness.org

Amblyopia (Lazy Eye)

DEREK HESS, M.D.

What Is It? · Amblyopia, or "lazy eye," is decreased vision in one or both eyes caused by disruption of normal visual development from a variety of causes during the first 7 to 9 years of life. Amblyopia affects about 3 of every 100 people and is a common cause of mild to severe visual loss.

Normal visual development in children may be impaired by one of three major factors and lead to amblyopia. First, strabismus, or eye misalignment, can cause amblyopia when a child "turns off" or ignores the image from one eye to avoid double vision. Second, refractive error, or needing glasses, can cause amblyopia, especially when there is a large difference in the refractive strength of the two eyes. Third, any blockage that prevents light from reaching the retina, such as a cloudy cornea, a cataract, or a droopy eyelid, can cause amblyopia. In all cases of amblyopia, if an eye is not used normally during childhood for prolonged periods, vision will not develop normally and can even permanently decrease.

Symptoms: What You May Experience · Adults with amblyopia since childhood have one eye that has poorer vision than the other, or poor vision in both eyes. Children with amblyopia may not notice poor vision in one eye. Parents of these children may notice crossing or drifting eyes, or whiteness of the pupil.

Examination Findings: What the Doctor Looks for · The eye doctor will evaluate any eye misalignment and white-looking pupils. However, amblyopia can sometimes be difficult to detect because it can lack obvious signs. Measuring the vision and the need for glasses and performing a complete eye exam to rule out other causes of decreased vision helps the eye doctor with the diagnosis.

What You Can Do · If you are an adult, nothing can be done to improve your amblyopia. If you are a parent of a child younger than 9 years old, you should ensure that your child undergoes vision screenings at school or at the pediatrician's office to detect amblyopia early so that treatment can be initiated.

When to Call the Doctor · If you are a parent of a young child, you should have your child examined by an eye doctor if you notice crossing or drifting eyes, a white-looking pupil, difficulty seeing, or any other eye abnormality.

Treatment · The treatment of amblyopia consists of making the child use the "lazy" eye. Usually this is accomplished by patching the good eye for much or all of the time. Atropine eye drops and special lenses can also be used to blur the good eye and thus encourage the child to use the amblyopic eye. If a cataract is present, surgical removal of the cataract may be required first before amblyopia can improve. Eye muscle surgery to correct eye misalignment may be done before or after patching therapy. In all cases, frequent follow-up visits with the eye doctor are necessary to monitor changes in vision.

Prognosis: Will I (or Will My Child) See Better? · Success in treating amblyopia depends on two factors: the severity of visual loss and the age at which therapy is started. The earlier amblyopia is diagnosed and treated, the more likely it is that vision will improve. Once vision has improved, maintenance therapy may be necessary until the child is past the amblyopic age (7–9 years old). Adult patients generally can no longer improve their amblyopic vision.

http://www.preventblindness.org/children/amblyopiaFAQ.html
http://www.nei.nih.gov/health/amblyopia/ http://www.aapos.org/

Orbital Cellulitis

PAUL S. RISKE, M.D.

What Is It? · Orbital cellulitis is an infection in the orbit, or eye socket, that can cause vision loss and serious systemic complications. Vision loss results from the increased pressure that the infection puts on the eyeball, its blood vessels, and the optic nerve. Orbital cellulitis is usually caused by a bacterial infection that spreads either from the sinuses or from an eyelid infection into the orbit. Sinus disease is the most common cause of orbital cellulitis because the sinuses are located next to the orbit, separated by a thin layer of bone. Serious sinus infections can spread through these orbital bones, some of which are paper-thin, to reach the orbit. In some cases of orbital cellulitis, an abscess, or pus collection, can form in the orbit.

Another cause of orbital cellulitis is infection of the eyelids and surrounding skin, which is called preseptal cellulitis. Although preseptal cellulitis can be severe, it is usually not vision threatening. However, if not treated promptly, this infection can sometimes penetrate the orbital septum, a thin layer of tissue behind the eyelids that normally helps prevent skin infections from reaching the orbit. Once the infection crosses this natural barrier, orbital cellulitis can result.

Symptoms: What You May Experience · Swelling of the eyelid, redness, and tenderness are early signs of preseptal or orbital cellulitis. There may be pus-like discharge from the eye, and a fever may or may not be present. Double vision, difficulty moving the eye, decreased vision, or an eye that bulges forward often signifies severe orbital involvement.

Examination Findings: What the Doctor Looks for · Your eye doctor will look for signs of infection in the eyelids and surrounding skin. He or she will check your vision, eye pressure, and eye position and movements. Your pupils may be dilated so that your optic nerves can be checked. A sample of pus-like discharge may be taken to find out what type of bacterium is causing the infection. When orbital cellulitis is suspected, blood tests and an imaging (computed tomography or CT) scan of the brain and orbits are often performed.

What You Can Do · If you have sinus disease or an eyelid infection, see your doctor to make sure these conditions are properly treated so that they do not result in orbital cellulitis.

When to Call the Doctor · If you notice eyelid swelling, redness, or tenderness, you should call your eye doctor. If you also have decreased vision, eye pain or discharge, double vision, difficulty moving the eye, or an eye that bulges forward, a doctor should examine you immediately.

Treatment · Orbital cellulitis is usually treated with hospitalization and intravenous antibiotics. If an abscess has formed or the orbital cellulitis is not responding to antibiotics, surgery may be required to drain the infection. Preseptal cellulitis is usually treated with oral antibiotics, and hospitalization may or may not be necessary, depending on the severity of the infection. Frequent monitoring of both these conditions is extremely important.

Prognosis: Will I See Better? · The prognosis of orbital cellulitis depends on the extent and severity of the infection. In many cases, your vision may return to normal after the infection resolves with proper treatment. If uncontrolled, however, the infection may spread beyond the orbit and reach the brain. Death is an extremely rare complication of orbital cellulitis.

http://www.nlm.nih.gov/medlineplus/ency/article/001012.htm
http://www.eyemdlink.com/Condition.asp?ConditionID=477

Tumors of the Orbit

THOMAS J. CUMMINGS, M.D.

What Is the Orbit? · The orbit is a complex region associated with seven bones and many soft tissues. These tissues include muscle, adipose tissue (fat), blood vessels, nerves, and the lacrimal gland, among others. All these elements have the potential to grow abnormally and form a tumor.

Which Tumors Involve the Orbit? · Tumors of the orbit can be either benign or malignant (cancerous). Common benign orbital tumors include hemangioma (tumor of the blood vessels), lymphangioma (tumor of lymphatics), lipoma (tumor of fat cells), and neurofibroma and schwannoma (tumors of nerve tissue). However, these cell types can also grow to form malignant tumors in some patients. Angiosarcoma and hemangiopericytoma are malignant blood vessel tumors, liposarcoma is a malignant tumor of fatty tissue, and malignant peripheral nerve sheath tumors can arise from originally benign neurofibromas in patients with diseases such as neurofibromatosis.

Malignant tumors of the orbit also include malignant tumors of muscle and meninges (the tissue that surrounds the optic nerve and the brain). Rhabdomyosarcoma is a malignant tumor that forms from skeletal muscle cells in children, while leiomyosarcoma is a malignant tumor of smooth muscle cells in adults. Orbital meningiomas are benign tumors of the meninges that surround the optic nerve along its path through the orbit to the brain. Benign and malignant tumors involving the bones and cartilage that protect the orbit can also occur.

Some tumors can involve both the orbit and the eye, or the orbit and the brain. Both retinoblastoma (a type of tumor inside the eyeball itself) and brain tumors can grow into the orbit. Lymphomas also can occur in the orbit because of the lymphoid tissue present there. The lacrimal gland can give rise to tumors that grow into the orbit, including the benign mixed tumor, also known as the pleomorphic adenoma, and the malignant adenoid cystic carcinoma, infamous for its tendency to spread along and invade nerves. Tumors of the orbit can affect vision by compressing and injuring the optic nerves or the muscles that move the eyeball.

In adults, the possibility that an orbital mass is metastatic, or has spread from another body part, must always be considered. These metastatic tumors can even be the first presenting sign of cancer in other parts of the body. The most common metastatic tumors to the orbit are from lung cancer and breast cancer, but they can spread from nearly any other site.

http://www.eyecancer.com/ http://www.eyecancerinfo.com

Orbital Ecchymosis (Black Eye)

HERB GREENMAN, M.D.

What Is It? · Orbital ecchymosis, or black eye, is a collection of fluid and blood in the tissues around the eye (orbit), leading to swelling and discoloration of the overlying eyelid skin. Orbital ecchymosis can be thought of as a bruising of tissues around the eye and is usually caused by trauma or surgery to the eyes, nose, or face. Rarely orbital ecchymosis can be caused by tumors, bleeding disorders, or blood-thinning medications.

Symptoms: What You May Experience · You may experience swelling and reddish discoloration of the eyelids and tissues surrounding the eye. The swelling may progress and may ultimately turn purple, yellow, green, or black.

Examination Findings: What the Doctor Looks for · The eye doctor will ask about any trauma to the eye and then look for any injury to the orbits such as a penetrating wound or orbital blow-out fracture. The doctor will perform a full eye exam, checking vision, eye pressure, and eye movements, and looking for injuries in and around the eye. Special x-rays may be performed to look for bony fractures or foreign objects.

What You Can Do · If the bruising is from a blunt eye injury, you can apply ice to your closed eyelids for 20 minutes every hour while awake for the first 24 hours after an injury to reduce the swelling. Do not apply ice or pressure to the eye if you think something pierced or entered your eyeball.

When to Call the Doctor · You should seek medical attention immediately if you think something pierced or entered the eye or if there are large cuts to the eye area. Symptoms of concern are decreased or double vision, loss of consciousness, blood or clear fluid from the nose or ears, blood on the surface of the eye, persistent headache, or severe pain. You should also see an eye doctor soon after an ecchymosis occurs if the swelling does not improve over several days, if the area of injury appears infected, or if the ecchymosis is not the result of an injury. In orbital ecchymosis due to an eye injury, you should follow up with an eye doctor even after the bruising has resolved, because you may be at risk for glaucoma or other eye problems.

Treatment · Treatment depends on the type of injuries incurred with a black eye. The black eye itself is normally treated with ice packs for the first 24 hours after the injury.

Prognosis: Will I See Better? · Over 1–2 weeks, the bruising of the skin will become lighter and the swelling will subside. The visual outcome depends on any associated eye injuries.

http://kidshealth.org/parent/firstaid_safe/emergencies/eye_injury.html
http://www.medem.com/medlb/article_detaillb.cfm?article_ID=
  ZZZEGMLPSKC&sub_cat=32

Hyphema

HERB GREENMAN, M.D.

What Is It? · A hyphema is blood in the anterior chamber. It may be caused by eye injury or eye surgery, or occur spontaneously. Spontaneous causes could include abnormal blood vessels growing on the iris, tumors in the eye, or bleeding disorders. Abnormal blood vessels on the iris may be triggered by lack of oxygen to the eye, diabetes, inflammation, or retinal detachment.

Symptoms: What You May Experience · You may have had a recent injury or surgery to your eye and now have sudden blurred vision and pain. The inside of the eyeball may appear to be partly or completely filled with blood.

Examination Findings: What the Doctor Looks for · The doctor will inquire about any recent eye injury. He or she will perform a com-

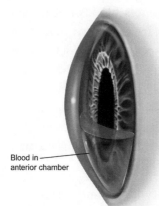

Blood in
anterior chamber

22 Blood fills the anterior
chamber in a hyphema.

plete eye exam, which will include looking for blood in the anterior chamber of your eye and checking your eye pressure. African Americans, Hispanics, and those of Mediterranean descent should be screened for sickle cell trait or disease, since patients with sickle cell are more likely to have permanent eye damage from a hyphema.

What You Can Do · Avoid eye injury to lessen your risk of developing a hyphema.

When to Call the Doctor · A hyphema is an eye emergency. You should be seen by an eye doctor as soon as possible.

Treatment · Cycloplegic (dilating) and steroid eye drops may be given to lessen inflammation in the eye, and pressure-lowering eye drops may be needed to control the eye pressure. You may be instructed to rest in bed with your head elevated as much as possible and to refrain from strenuous activity and from taking blood-thinning medications. Rarely patients, particularly children, may need to be admitted to the hospital.

Much of the time, the blood will be naturally reabsorbed by your body. However, surgery to remove the blood clot may be indicated if the hyphema is large and lasts for more than 5–10 days, if the cornea is stained by blood, or if the eye pressure cannot be controlled with medications.

Prognosis: Will I See Better? · In many cases the vision will improve as the hyphema resolves. If the eye pressure was extremely high for a very long time when the hyphema occurred, the optic nerve could be damaged by the pressure, which may affect your vision. In cases of blunt eye injury, how much vision is ultimately restored usually depends on the extent of the initial injuries. The status of your retina may also be a determining factor in the outcome, especially in cases of spontaneous hyphema.

http://www.emedicine.com/oph/topic142.htm
http://www.nlm.nih.gov/medlineplus/ency/article/001021.htm

Orbital Blow-out Fracture

KENNETH NEUFELD, M.D. · JULIE A. WOODWARD, M.D.

What Is It? · An orbital blow-out fracture is a fracture (broken bone) of one or more of the bony walls of the orbit, which is the "eye socket" where the eyeball rests. When a large object strikes the eye, forces are transmitted through the orbit, which cause the bones to break and literally "blow out" into the surrounding sinuses. Of the four sides of bone in the orbit, the medial side wall (next to the nose) and the bottom wall (known as the orbital floor) are the weakest and therefore most commonly sustain blow-out fractures.

Symptoms: What You May Experience · If you have had a blunt injury to your eye and developed an orbital blow-out fracture, you may have face or eye pain, swelling, bruising, and possibly a nosebleed. The affected eye may have restricted movement, especially when you try to look up or down, which can cause double vision. There may be numbness of the cheek, upper lip, or teeth on the affected side. These symptoms occur because a muscle or nerve may be pinched in the fracture. The eye may have a sunken position relative to the other, unaffected eye.

Examination Findings: What the Doctor Looks for · Besides checking for injuries in other parts of your body, your doctor will check your vision and eye movements. Your eyes will also be examined to see if the eyeball itself has been injured. If an orbital blow-out fracture is suspected, an imaging scan such as a computed tomography, or CT, scan may be done.

What You Can Do · The best way to avoid an orbital blow-out fracture is to avoid blunt eye injury. Use protective eyewear in situations where eye injury is possible.

When to Call the Doctor · If you have been hit in the eye, you should seek medical attention at your closest emergency room as soon as possible.

Treatment · In most cases patients with a diagnosed orbital blow-out fracture should apply ice packs to the face and eye as often as tolerated for the first 48 hours. They should avoid blowing their nose and may be prescribed a nasal decongestant spray and oral antibiotics.

An orbital blow-out fracture often does not need to be surgically repaired immediately, since swelling, bleeding, and double vision may resolve spontaneously after 10 to 14 days. Some small fractures do not need surgery at all. Usually optimal surgical repair is accomplished within the first 2 weeks after the injury. Signs that do warrant more urgent surgery include double vision in straight-ahead or downward gaze; a sunken position of the eyeball of 2 mm or greater relative to the other, unaffected eye; or a slowed heart rate caused by the eye injury, which will rarely occur. In repairing the fracture, the surgeon will attempt to remove any tissues trapped within the fracture and to place a new orbital wall, which may be made of bone or synthetic material, against the fractured wall.

You should see your eye doctor periodically after this type of injury to make sure that the fracture heals properly and that no late complications, such as double vision or glaucoma, develop.

Prognosis: Will I See Better? · The prognosis for vision and facial appearance depends on the extent of the initial injury. Many patients recover extremely well after treatment.

http://www.asoprs.org/Pages/trauma.html

http://www.medem.com/medlb/article_detaillb.cfm?article_ID=
ZZZ5JXSWIOC&sub_cat=32

Open Globe

PAUL KANG, M.D.

What Is It? · An open globe occurs when the eyeball is cut open
or ruptures open. This can occur from any type of injury to the
eye from a variety of sources (such as rocks, bottles, motor ve-
hicle accidents, fists, and sporting injuries). There can be many
other problems associated with an open globe, including cataract,
bleeding, glaucoma, retinal detachment, or foreign objects inside
the eyeball (called intraocular foreign bodies).

Symptoms: What You May Experience · Patients usually have a history of eye injury and resulting pain and profound decrease in
vision. They may also notice a deformity in the normal shape of
the eyeball.

Examination Findings: What the Doctor Looks for · The doctor looks
for a full-thickness wound or hole in the eye as well as any possible
foreign body. Through careful examination, the ophthalmologist
may find low eye pressure, eye deformity, eyeball contents outside
the eye, and bleeding. A computed tomography (CT) scan of the
eye area may be obtained to search for a foreign body in or around
the eye.

What You Can Do · It is best to avoid eye injury if at all possible.
Wear eye protection whenever participating in high-risk activities.
If an open globe does occur, go to the nearest emergency room
right away. Tape a plastic cup over the eye (open end toward the
face) to protect it, taking care not to touch or put any pressure on
the eye. Try not to cough, sneeze, or do anything to increase pressure to your head. Do not eat or drink anything after the injury
in case emergency surgery must be performed.

When to Call the Doctor · Once you experience eye injury and suspect eye damage, go to the nearest emergency room right away.

Treatment · The goal of treating an open globe is to surgically close the wound, thus stabilizing the eye and preventing infection and complications. If an intraocular foreign body is present, this must also be removed. Emergency surgery is performed, usually within 24–48 hours. Intravenous antibiotics may be given before or during surgery. After surgery, eye drops and medications may be prescribed to prevent infection, control eye inflammation and pressure, and make the eye feel more comfortable. Even if initial surgery to close the wound is successful, future operations are often necessary to treat the complications that accompany this type of injury.

Prognosis: Will I See Better? · Usually ophthalmologists are successful in closing the eye wound. The final visual outcome varies widely and depends on the extent of the initial injury. Sometimes the eye is injured so much that it is not repairable and must be removed.

http://www.medem.com/medlb/article_detaillb.cfm?article_ID=
ZZZCAQQWIOC&sub_cat=32
http://kidshealth.org/parent/firstaid_safe/emergencies/
eye_injury.html

Foreign Body

PAUL KANG, M.D.

What Is It? · A foreign body is any object in or on the eye that is not naturally there. A surface foreign body is on the outside of the eyeball, whereas an intraocular foreign body is inside the eyeball. Intraocular foreign bodies were discussed in the immediately preceding section on "open globe" injuries; surface foreign bodies will be discussed here. These can be anything from a piece of wood or metal to an insect or a piece of torn contact lens. Foreign bodies can cause eye discomfort, and if not removed may lead to infection or other problems.

Symptoms: What You May Experience · Persons with a corneal or conjunctival foreign body may feel as if there is something scratching their eye. They may have eye pain, tearing, redness, and sensitivity to light. They may remember that an object flew into their eye.

Examination Findings: What the Doctor Looks for · The doctor looks for the foreign body itself to determine whether it is on the surface of the eyeball or actually inside the eye. An intraocular foreign body is much more serious and requires prompt surgical removal. To see the foreign body the eye doctor may use a special fluorescent eye drop and a slit lamp. He or she may also flip the upper eyelids to ensure that nothing is hidden under them. If a foreign body is suspected but not found on thorough examination, an ultrasound or a computed tomography (CT) scan of the eyes may also be performed.

What You Can Do · Prevention is critical. Always wear eye protection when there is a possibility that a foreign substance will come into contact with the eye. If something does enter the eye, try to remove it by gently flushing the eye with clean water. Avoid rubbing or pressing on the eye.

When to Call the Doctor · If you are unable to remove the foreign body with gentle flushing, call the doctor immediately.

Treatment · The doctor will find and remove the foreign body. He or she may also prescribe an antibiotic eye drop or ointment afterward to help the eye heal.

Prognosis: Will I See Better? · Once a surface foreign body is removed, the eye generally heals well and feels more comfortable. The final visual outcome depends largely on the size and location of the foreign body as well as the extent of the initial injury.

http://www.medem.com/medlb/article_detaillb.cfm?article_ID= ZZZCAQQWIOC&sub_cat=2015

http://www.medem.com/medlb/article_detaillb.cfm?article_ID= ZZZFDIAP3SC&sub_cat=2015

Chemical Injury

PAUL KANG, M.D.

What Is It? · A chemical injury can occur when a chemical is splashed onto the eye. Common sources of injury are household cleaners, fertilizers, or industrial chemicals used on the job. Some cases can be potentially blinding. Although both acid and alkali chemicals can cause eye injury, alkali injuries tend to be especially severe.

Symptoms: What You May Experience · After a chemical splash to the eye, patients may experience eye pain, redness, tearing, light sensitivity, and possibly decreased vision.

Examination Findings: What the Doctor Looks for · If a chemical injury is suspected, a doctor will flush the eye with saline solution before even examining it. Afterward the doctor will assess the amount of injury that the chemical may have caused. He or she may also check the eye's pH and look for any residual chemical particles to make sure that none remain in the eye.

What You Can Do · Always wear eye protection when working with chemicals that may splash into your eyes. If a chemical does enter your eye, ask someone else to call 911 and IMMEDIATELY begin constant flushing of the eyes with clean water, in a shower or using an eye wash station, until 911 help arrives.

When to Call the Doctor · After you have asked someone to call 911 and immediately flushed your eyes with clean water, seek medical attention promptly. Bring the bottle of the material that splashed into your eye to the doctor.

Treatment · The treatment of a chemical eye injury is to flush out the chemical in the eye. Further treatment depends on the extent of the injury and may include antibiotic and lubricating eye drops or even eye surgery in the future.

Prognosis: Will I See Better? · The final visual outcome depends on the extent of the injury, the type of chemical, and how long the chemical was in the eye before removal. Many patients with mild chemical eye injuries improve markedly after the chemicals are removed from the eye.

http://www.aapcc.org/facsheets/parentfactsheet.PDF
http://www.medem.com/medlb/article_detaillb.cfm?article_ID= ZZZCAQQWIOC&sub_cat=32

Eyelid Lacerations

PAUL S. RISKE, M.D.

What Is It? · An eyelid laceration is a wound on the eyelid, often caused by an injury. Because of the eyelids' role in protecting and lubricating the eyeball, special consideration should be given to treating and repairing the laceration. Important considerations include protecting the cornea, maintaining proper eyelid motion, and cosmetic appearance.

Symptoms: What You May Experience · After an eyelid injury, you may notice a wound on the eyelid. If the tear drainage system has been damaged, excessive eye watering can occur.

Examination Findings: What the Doctor Looks for · As part of a thorough eye exam to rule out any other eye injury, your eye doctor will examine your eyelid for a laceration. He or she will see if the laceration involves the edge of the eyelid or the tear drainage system, which may require probing of the tear duct with a small metal rod.

What You Can Do · The best way to avoid an eyelid laceration is to avoid eye injury. If your eyelid or eyeball is injured, seek medical attention immediately and do not touch the eye.

When to Call the Doctor · If your eyelids are injured, go to the emergency room or see an eye doctor promptly.

Treatment · Most eyelid lacerations should be repaired within 48 hours of the injury. Surface lacerations that only involve the skin may be repaired with stitches in the emergency room or office under local anesthetic and do not usually require extensive surgery in the operating room. Antibiotic ointment is then prescribed for the wound, and the stitches are usually removed in 7–14 days. Lacerations that run through the edge of the eyelid require more complicated stitches to ensure correct alignment and prevent an indentation along the edge of the eyelid, which could cause problems with tearing, incomplete closure, and irritation to the cornea.

Eyelid lacerations that occur at the innermost corner of the eyelids, toward the nose, may potentially disrupt the tear drainage system and result in excessive eye watering. A laceration that involves this drainage system may require more extensive surgery in the operating room. A silicone tube may be placed in the drainage system during the surgery to ensure that the drainage channels do not scar shut as the wound heals. The tube is normally removed after 3–6 months.

Prognosis: Will I See Better? · Many properly repaired eyelid lacerations heal well with minimal scarring. However, if significant scarring of the eyelid develops, the eyelid may turn outward and cause tearing and irritation to the cornea, or it may turn inward, causing the eyelashes to rub against the eyeball. Scarring of the tear drainage system and the excessive eye watering that results will sometimes occur despite proper placement of the tube. This sort of scarring may require further eyelid surgery.

http://www.mdadvice.com/library/sport/sport257.html
http://www.emedicine.com/oph/topic219.htm

Ocular Prosthesis (Artificial or Glass Eye)

KENNETH NEUFELD, M.D. · JULIE A. WOODWARD, M.D.

What Is an Ocular Prosthesis? · An ocular prosthesis is a medical term for an artificial eyeball. Until the 1950s most ocular prostheses were made of glass. Today it is more common to use acrylic. Current ocular prostheses are crafted and painted by specialists known as ocularists and look almost identical to real eyes.

The prosthetic eye does not give any vision. It is used to resemble a "normal" eye and maintain the volume of the eye socket.

The part of the prosthesis that is visible is called a shell. This shell can be placed over a sick eye, a shrunken eye, or most commonly an implant. An implant is a sphere made of plastic, silicone, or hydroxyapatite (a material derived from sea coral) which is surgically placed in the orbit at the time a sick eye is removed and is meant to stay in permanently. It is needed to replace orbital volume and provide eye movement for the prosthesis. The patient will be able to move the prosthetic eye somewhat, but probably not as easily as the other, "normal" eye. Motility can sometimes be improved if a connecting peg is placed in the implant and connected to the overlying shell.

Why Are Ocular Protheses Needed? · People may have prosthetic eyes for a variety of reasons. The most common reason to remove a natural, blind eye is to relieve pain. The blind, painful eye is replaced with a prosthetic eye, which usually is completely pain free. In other cases a natural eye sustains severe injury, cannot be salvaged, and may need to be removed to decrease the risk of a very rare condition called sympathetic ophthalmia, which can cause visual loss in the good eye. Other patients may be born with congenital abnormalities requiring the use of a prosthetic eye. If cancer is detected in an eye or surrounding orbit, the treatment may involve removal of the affected eye to decrease the likelihood that the cancer will spread.

When Is an Ocular Prosthesis Placed? · After a natural eye is removed for any of the above reasons, the tissues in the orbit need time to heal and become strong enough to hold the prosthetic shell over the implant. Once the tissues heal well without exposure of the implant, then the patient may have a prosthetic shell custom fitted. This usually occurs about 6 weeks after surgery.

Living with an Ocular Prosthesis · After the shell has been fitted, very little maintenance is necessary. The prosthetic shell should be cleaned approximately once a week as directed by your eye doctor. He or she will examine the eye socket periodically to make sure that the tissues over the implant remain healed. The prosthetic shell should be polished by an ocularist once a year. In most cases, patients are extremely satisfied with their ocular prostheses and can live a relatively normal life.

http://www.eyemdlink.com/EyeProcedure.asp?EyeProcedureID=35
http://www.ocularists.org/index.html

15 · Systemic Diseases That Affect Vision and the Eye

Diabetes Mellitus

KELLY WALTON MUIR, M.D.

What Is It? · Diabetes mellitus is a disease of abnormal blood sugar regulation. Type 1 diabetes often occurs in children and is characterized by the body's inability to make insulin, which the body needs to properly use the sugar in the blood. Although there is some overlap between the affected populations, type 2 diabetes occurs primarily in adults: in type 2 diabetes the body does make insulin but is resistant to it. Diabetes, especially type 2, often runs in families.

Symptoms: What You May Experience · When the blood sugar is abnormally high, the lens in the eye may swell, causing blurred vision. The eye doctor may be the first person to suspect that the patient has diabetes because the patient's eyeglass prescription keeps changing as the blood sugar goes up and down. Long-standing diabetes can cause permanent damage throughout the body, including the eyes. In fact, diabetes is the most common cause of blindness in adults in the United States.

Examination Findings: What the Doctor Looks for · Diabetes can cause abnormalities throughout the eye. Your eye doctor will look for problems in the cornea, early-onset cataracts, bleeding in the retina, and the growth of abnormal blood vessels.

What You Can Do · Research studies have shown that controlling blood sugar can prevent the long-term complications of diabetes in your eyes and throughout your body. Your primary care doctor or endocrinologist can help you develop a diet and exercise plan and possibly recommend medications to keep your blood sugar within the normal range.

When to Call the Doctor · Blurred vision in both eyes together, increased thirst, urinary frequency, and unexplained weight loss are all suggestive of diabetes and should prompt you to call your doctors. If you have been recently diagnosed with diabetes, you should have a complete eye exam as soon as possible. Subsequent eye exams will be scheduled based on your current eye exam findings. You could have diabetic damage in the eye without experiencing any symptoms, so routine exams are important.

Treatment · If complications of diabetes develop in the eye, your eye doctor may recommend laser treatment or eye surgery to prevent further visual loss.

Prognosis: Will I See Better? · With appropriate blood sugar control and regular eye exams, people with diabetes may never experience any change in vision. However, long-standing high blood sugar can lead to irreversible visual loss and even blindness.

http://www.diabetes.org/homepage.jsp
http://www.nlm.nih.gov/medlineplus/ency/article/001214.htm

Hypertension (High Blood Pressure)

KELLY WALTON MUIR, M.D.

What Is It? · Hypertension, or high blood pressure, is one of the most common chronic diseases in the United States. In most cases the exact cause is unknown, but hypertension occurs more frequently with advanced age and sometimes runs in families.

Symptoms: What You May Experience · One reason why hypertension is a difficult disease to treat is that there are usually no symptoms. People can have hypertension for many years without knowing it, until they experience one of the long-term complications of the disease. These complications include stroke, kidney damage, heart failure, and retinopathy (damage to the retina). Blurred vision may be a sign of hypertensive retinopathy.

Examination Findings: What the Doctor Looks for · Your doctor will do a complete eye exam to evaluate for bleeding in the retina, blocked blood vessels, or signs of damage to the nerves or the retina.

What You Can Do · Maintaining your blood pressure within the normal range can prevent the ocular complications of hypertension. Your primary care doctor can help you to achieve good blood pressure control with proper diet, exercise, and possibly medications.

When to Call the Doctor · Although chronic hypertension usually does not cause any symptoms, when the blood pressure becomes extremely high one may develop blurred vision, headache, or blood in the urine. Even without visual problems, people with hypertension should have a complete eye exam once a year to evaluate for retinopathy.

Treatment · The treatment of hypertensive eye disease is controlling the blood pressure.

Prognosis: Will I See Better? · Most people with hypertension will not experience permanent visual loss from hypertension alone, but high blood pressure is a risk factor for other eye diseases that often lead to irreversible loss of vision. Such diseases include age-related macular degeneration and retinal vascular occlusions.

http://www.americanheart.org/presenter.jhtml?identifier=2114
http://www.nhlbi.nih.gov/hbp/index.html

Hyperthyroidism and Graves Disease

JENNIFER S. WEIZER, M.D. · JOHN J. MICHON, M.D.

What Is It? · Hyperthyroidism is a condition in which the thyroid gland, located in the neck, is overactive and secretes too much thyroid hormone. Graves disease, the most common cause of hyperthyroidism, is an autoimmune disease of unknown origin which makes the thyroid gland overactive. Thyroid eye disease is a set of typical problems associated with thyroid dysfunction that affects one or both eyes. Usually an overactive thyroid gland from Graves disease causes the eye problems, but in some cases an underactive thyroid or a thyroid that secretes normal amounts of its hormone can be associated with this eye disorder. Thyroid eye disease can sometimes persist even when thyroid hormone levels are corrected with treatment, and women are more often affected than men.

Typical eye findings in thyroid eye disease include bulging eyes, upper and lower eyelids pulling backward so that the eyelids do not cover enough of the eyeball, dry eye syndrome, double vision from strabismus caused by inflammation of the eye muscles, and optic nerve damage (optic neuropathy).

Symptoms: What You May Experience · You may notice eye redness, irritation, double vision, decreased vision, difficulty distinguishing colors, bulging of one or both eyes, or a pulling backward of the upper or lower eyelids so that the top and bottom white parts of your eyeball are abnormally visible.

Examination Findings: What the Doctor Looks for · Your eye doctor will check your vision, pupils, eye pressure (sometimes while you look upward as well as straight ahead), color vision, eye movements, and general eye appearance. The front part of your eyeballs will be examined with a slit lamp for inflammation and signs of dry eye from poor eyelid closure. Your eye doctor may measure how far your eyes bulge forward, and your pupils will be dilated so that your optic nerves can be examined. You may be asked to perform a test for peripheral, or side, vision.

If your eye doctor suspects thyroid eye disease as a cause of your symptoms, he or she may order a special x-ray (CT or MRI) to look at your eye muscles and optic nerve within the orbit. In thyroid eye disease, the eye muscles may be swollen and enlarged and may compress the optic nerve.

What You Can Do · There is no proven way to avoid the development of hyperthyroidism. If you have thyroid disease, controlling your thyroid hormone levels with the help of your medical doctor may help to prevent or alleviate the eye complications of the disease.

When to Call the Doctor · If you notice sustained eye redness, irritation, double vision, decreased vision, difficulty distinguishing colors, bulging of one or both eyes, or a pulling backward of your upper or lower eyelids so that the top and bottom white parts of your eyeball are abnormally visible, call your eye doctor. Prompt treatment can sometimes lessen the permanent damage caused by severe thyroid eye disease.

Treatment · Many people with mild thyroid eye disease only require artificial tears or lubricating ointment to help with their dry eye symptoms. Normalizing your thyroid hormone levels with the help of your medical doctor is important and usually helps to stabilize the eye disease. Severe flares of inflammation in thyroid eye disease that threaten to dry out the cornea or damage the optic nerve can sometimes be treated with oral steroid medications, radiation therapy, or surgery to decompress the orbit and provide space for the inflamed tissues.

Once thyroid eye disease has stabilized for at least several months and the inflammation is controlled, surgery to correct any remaining problems with eyelid position or strabismus can be considered with your ophthalmologist. Prescribing prisms in eyeglasses often helps to correct stable double vision caused by thyroid eye disease.

Prognosis: Will I See Better? · The prognosis for thyroid eye disease depends largely on the severity of the eye problems. Permanent optic nerve damage is relatively rare, thus preserving most patients' level of vision. The appearance of the eyes and double vision are typically the most serious issues for persons with thyroid eye disease, but fortunately treatments for these problems are often successful.

http://thyroid.about.com/ http://www.asoprs.org/Pages/thyroid.html

Multiple Sclerosis

KELLY WALTON MUIR, M.D.

What Is It? · Multiple sclerosis is a disease of the brain and spinal cord in which the body attacks its own central nervous system and causes neurological problems. The cause of multiple sclerosis is unknown, but it occurs more commonly in women than men and more often in Caucasians than African Americans. The optic nerves (in optic neuritis) and the parts of the brain that control eye movements are sometimes affected in multiple sclerosis. Rarely, multiple sclerosis can cause inflammation inside the eye (pars planitis).

Symptoms: What You May Experience · The symptoms of multiple sclerosis vary greatly. People with multiple sclerosis may experience weakness or numbness in an arm or leg, double vision, decreased vision, or an abnormal blind spot. Some people have only a few attacks, and some people have many attacks over their lifetime.

Examination Findings: What the Doctor Looks for · Your eye doctor will measure your vision, test eye movements, and look for an abnormal blind spot. Many people with multiple sclerosis will have a completely normal eye exam, but abnormalities in vision or eye alignment may cause your doctor to consider the possibility of multiple sclerosis. If your eye doctor or neurologist is concerned about multiple sclerosis, he or she may order a magnetic resonance imaging (MRI) study to evaluate the brain for damage.

What You Can Do · There is no known prevention for multiple sclerosis.

When to Call the Doctor · If you experience weakness or numbness, you should call your primary care doctor or neurologist. If you experience double vision, decreased vision, or a blind spot in your vision, you should call your eye doctor. If you have multiple sclerosis, you should have annual eye exams to ensure that your eyes are not affected by the disease.

Treatment · There are several new treatment options for multiple sclerosis, including intravenous steroids and other medicines which help control the immune system. Your eye doctor, neurologist, or primary care doctor can help you decide which might be best for you.

Prognosis: Will I See Better? · Most of the time, when an eye attack of multiple sclerosis resolves, the vision returns to normal and any double vision goes away. In some circumstances, however, visual loss can be permanent.

http://www.nationalmssociety.org/ **http:**//www.msfacts.org/

Autoimmune Diseases

KELLY WALTON MUIR, M.D.

What Is It? · A variety of diseases are categorized as autoimmune. The exact causes of these diseases are unknown, but all involve a malfunction of the body's immune system. Diseases in this category include systemic lupus erythematosus, rheumatoid arthritis, sarcoidosis, ankylosing spondylitis, and Sjogren's syndrome.

Symptoms: What You May Experience · Each of the autoimmune diseases can have multiple effects on the eye. Dry eye syndrome is common to many of the autoimmune diseases, particularly Sjogren's syndrome. Inflammation of the eye, such as in uveitis, scleritis, and episcleritis, may be caused by these diseases when the body's immune system begins to attack the eye. Inflammation of the eye may cause eye pain, decreased vision, and a red eye.

Examination Findings: What the Doctor Looks for · Inflammation of the eye without a known cause may lead your doctor to suspect an autoimmune disease. The optic nerve, retinal blood vessels, or cornea may all show signs of inflammation in some of the autoimmune diseases.

What You Can Do · There is no known prevention for autoimmune diseases. Tell your doctor if you have a family history of autoimmune disease, as this may increase your own risk of developing such a disease.

When to Call the Doctor · If you experience decreased vision or eye pain you should call your doctor. If you have an autoimmune disease, you should undergo a complete eye exam once a year. Some of the medications used to treat autoimmune diseases, such as steroids, can cause problems in the eye, such as glaucoma and cataract, so if you are taking medication for an autoimmune disease, you should ask your doctor if you need to be monitored with regular eye exams.

Treatment · Autoimmune diseases are often treated with steroids, which can be taken by mouth or as eye drops. There are also many new treatments (immunosuppressive medications) that target the immune system in much the same way as steroids but have different side effects.

Prognosis: Will I See Better? · Most people with autoimmune diseases never experience any visual problems, but in certain situations permanent visual loss (often caused by long-standing inflammation in the eye) may occur. Your eye doctor can tell you what to expect depending on your individual situation.

http://www.aarda.org/

Migraine

KELLY WALTON MUIR, M.D.

What Is It? · A migraine is an attack of neurologic or mood disturbance which often, but not always, includes headache. Migraines are more common in women and are experienced by as many as 34% of women aged 15–20. Most patients who suffer from migraines experience recurrent attacks, but the frequency of attacks is different for each person. No one is certain what causes migraines, but the disorder often runs in families.

Symptoms: What You May Experience · The typical migraine headache affects one side of the head at a time and may cause nausea or vomiting. Many people experience an unusual sensation called an "aura" before the onset of the headache, which may include a particular smell, sound, or visual change. A common visual change with migraine is a zigzag pattern in your vision which flickers and expands. Occasionally the "aura" is not followed by a headache. This is called an ophthalmic migraine.

Examination Findings: What the Doctor Looks for · The eye exam is almost always normal in people with migraines, but in rare circumstances the doctor can detect an abnormal blind spot or a misalignment of the eyes. These problems usually resolve with time (over days to weeks).

What You Can Do · If you experience migraines, it may help to keep track of what you eat and drink and when the migraines occur. Some people find that eliminating foods like chocolate or alcohol from their diet can prevent migraine attacks.

When to Call the Doctor · If you begin to have new, severe headaches, you should tell your primary care doctor so that he or she can determine the cause. Other diseases besides migraine can cause flickering lights or an abnormal blind spot, so if you experience these visual changes you should see your eye doctor.

Treatment · There are many new medications to prevent recurrent migraines and treat attacks when they happen. Your primary medical doctor can help you decide which one is best for you.

Prognosis: Will I See Better? · The visual changes associated with migraines almost always resolve in minutes to hours.

http://www.eyemdlink.com/condition.asp?conditionID=288
http://www.emedicinehealth.com/articles/9385-1.asp

Temporal (Giant Cell) Arteritis

DAVID A. CHESNUTT, M.D.

What Is It? · Temporal arteritis, also known as giant cell arteritis, is an inflammatory disease of the blood vessels. When blood vessels become inflamed, they are not able to carry the normal amount of blood to supply the body's tissues, which can lead to tissue damage. Temporal arteritis can affect many parts of the body, but the optic nerves are one of the most commonly affected sites. When the blood supply to the optic nerves is inadequate, optic neuropathy can result, leading to vision loss. Temporal arteritis is usually only seen in people older than 55 years of age and is slightly more common in women than men.

Symptoms: What You May Experience · If you have temporal arteritis, you may experience sudden vision loss in one or both eyes. Less commonly, you may notice double vision. However, vision problems are usually not the first symptom of temporal arteritis. Other common symptoms which may precede visual changes include severe headache, scalp tenderness (particularly at the temples), shoulder and hip aches, weight loss, poor appetite, fatigue, fever, or jaw pain when chewing.

Examination Findings: What the Doctor Looks for · Your eye doctor will perform a complete eye exam, looking for other causes of vision loss or double vision. He or she will ask about the symptoms of temporal arteritis and touch the skin covering the blood vessels near your temples, since these may be tender and inflamed in this disease. If temporal arteritis is suspected, blood tests to look for inflammation may be performed. The most definitive test to diagnose temporal arteritis is a biopsy of the temporal artery. In this surgical procedure, your ophthalmologist takes a small sample of a blood vessel in the temple area of the head, to be examined for inflammation under a microscope.

What You Can Do · There is no known way to prevent temporal arteritis from occurring.

When to Call the Doctor · If you experience vision loss or double vision, especially if accompanied by severe headache, scalp tenderness (particularly at the temples), shoulder and hip aches, weight loss, poor appetite, fatigue, fever, or jaw pain when chewing, see your eye doctor immediately. Prompt diagnosis of this disease is the key to preserving vision. Severe visual loss may occur in one or both eyes if the disease is left untreated even for a few days.

Treatment · Since temporal arteritis is an inflammatory condition, the main treatment consists of anti-inflammatory medications, such as steroids, which are usually given by mouth and do not require the patient to be hospitalized. Treatment is often started before the diagnosis is confirmed by temporal artery biopsy. Most patients with temporal arteritis will need to take anti-inflammatory medication for 18–24 months. The long-term side effects of taking steroid medication for this amount of time are lessened by gradually reducing the dose over the course of treatment. In patients who have significant steroid side effects, other anti-inflammatory medicines, such as methotrexate, may be used along with or instead of steroids.

Prognosis: Will I See Better? · The goal of treating temporal arteritis is to prevent vision loss in the other eye and other tissue damage throughout the body from the blood vessel inflammation. Anti-inflammatory treatment is generally effective in preventing further damage from the disease, so diagnosing and treating temporal arteritis promptly is extremely important. The vision loss that occurred before the start of treatment is often severe and permanent.

http://www.aafp.org/afp/20000815/789.html
http://www.ninds.nih.gov/health_and_medical/disorders/
vasculitis_doc.htm **http:**//www.aafp.org/afp/20000415/tips/6.html

Sexually Transmitted Diseases

KELLY WALTON MUIR, M.D.

What Is It? · Many sexually transmitted diseases can affect the eye. These include human immunodeficiency virus (HIV), gonorrhea, chlamydia, herpes, human papilloma virus, and syphilis. These diseases act differently from one another, but all can cause inflammation in or around the eye.

Symptoms: What You May Experience · Gonorrhea causes a conjunctivitis, or inflammation of the conjunctiva, characterized by lots of pus-like discharge from the eye. Chlamydia also causes conjunctivitis, but in chlamydial conjunctivitis there is less discharge and the inflammation may be long-standing. Human papilloma virus causes warts on the eyelids or eyeball. Herpes viruses and syphilis can cause corneal infections or inflammation (uveitis) inside the eye, leading to eye pain and decreased vision.

Examination Findings: What the Doctor Looks for · Your doctor will look for discharge from the eye, abnormalities of the cornea or conjunctiva, and inflammation inside the eye. If the exam suggests a sexually transmitted disease, he or she may recommend blood tests or take a sample of the infected area and send it to the laboratory for analysis.

What You Can Do · The only guaranteed prevention for sexually transmitted diseases is abstinence. The use of condoms decreases the risk of getting a sexually transmitted disease.

When to Call the Doctor · If you experience eye pain, decreased vision, or a red eye, you should call your eye doctor to be evaluated for an infection.

Treatment · There is systemic treatment available for all sexually transmitted diseases, but not all can be cured. The best treatment is prevention.

Prognosis: Will I See Better? · With appropriate treatment, most people with sexually transmitted diseases do not lose vision, but some eye infections can be very serious. For instance, conjunctivitis caused by gonorrhea can damage the eye very rapidly if not recognized and treated. Herpes and syphilis can cause irreversible damage to many parts of the eye.

http://www.niaid.nih.gov/factsheets/stdinfo.htm
http://www.medem.com/medlb/article_detaillb.cfm?article_ID=
　ZZZO6I53AKC&sub_cat=292

Brain Tumors

THOMAS J. CUMMINGS, M.D.

Some Facts about Brain Tumors · Brain tumors are known to occur across all age groups, from infants to the elderly. There are many types of brain tumors, some benign and others malignant, or cancerous. Some arise from the cells of the brain tissue, and others arise from the meninges (the layers of tissue that cover and protect the brain) or skull bones. The diagnosis is usually suspected in a person with neurological signs and symptoms, localized by special x-rays including CT scan and MRI, and ultimately confirmed by the surgeon removing the tumor and the pathologist classifying its cell type after looking at it under the microscope.

How Do Brain Tumors Affect Vision? · Brain tumors can affect vision in many ways, depending on their size, location, and cell type. Vision is a complex function that involves the eye and brain. The eyes and brain are connected by the optic nerves (the nerves necessary for vision), and the visual system extends to the occipital lobe (the part of the brain located at the back of the head). As brain tumors increase in size, the pressure within the skull (intracranial pressure) increases, compressing the brain. This can result in swelling of the optic nerve heads where they leave the eyeball (papilledema), a finding that can be made by an ophthalmologist or other physician during eye examination. Long-standing elevations in intracranial pressure can result in atrophy, or permanent damage, of the optic nerves. Vision can also be altered by tumors growing within the visual pathway that disrupt the flow of signals from the eyeball back to the brain, or by tumors that damage brain nerves involved in moving the eyeball.

What Are Some Common Examples of Brain Tumors that Can Affect Vision? · *Optic nerve astrocytomas.* Astrocytes are cells normally found in brain tissue that serve a supporting role for the brain and can be thought of as servants to maintain the health of the neurons (the cells of the brain required for intelligence and higher functions). Astrocytomas are tumors of astrocytes that are usually slow-growing and benign in childhood but malignant in adults. Astrocytomas can grow directly from the optic nerves, or the optic nerves can be affected by astrocytomas or other primary brain tumors that begin in the brain and grow into the nerves secondarily.

Pituitary adenomas. The pituitary gland is a small organ located beneath the optic chiasm (which is part of the visual pathway) at the base of the brain. Abnormal growth of the pituitary cells responsible for hormonal function can produce tumors that extend upward and compress the optic chiasm, usually resulting in loss of peripheral vision in both eyes.

Meningiomas. The meninges are three layers of tissue that cover and protect the brain within the skull. Tumors of the meninges can grow slowly to large sizes. They affect vision by taking up space within the skull, which raises intracranial pressure and compresses the optic nerves, or by directly compressing other nerves necessary for vision.

Pineal gland tumors. The pineal gland is a small gland located close to the center of the brain. It is responsible for the sleep-wake cycle and is sometimes thought of as the "third eye" because it is developmentally related to the retina. Pineal gland tumors can result in Parinaud's syndrome, with dilated pupils and difficulty looking upward.

Metastatic tumors. The most common brain tumors are those that travel to the brain from other body sites. Nearly all cancers can metastasize to the brain, and the more common ones include cancers of the lung, breast, kidney, and intestine, and melanomas. They often metastasize to the occipital lobe, where they can disrupt the function of the visual system.

http://cancer.duke.edu/btc/ http://www.abta.org/

Stroke and Cranial Nerve Palsies

DAVID A. CHESNUTT, M.D.

What Is It? · Stroke refers to damage to brain tissue from a sudden lack of blood supply. Risk factors for stroke include high blood pressure and smoking. When stroke damages the visual centers in the brain, a number of problems can result. One such problem involves the specialized nerves, called cranial nerves, which help to control and coordinate eye movements and eye alignment. Other parts of the brain which can be damaged by stroke include the areas that control peripheral, or side, vision.

Symptoms: What You May Experience · Persons with cranial nerve problems due to stroke may notice the sudden onset of double vision because both eyes are no longer properly aligned together. This double vision typically disappears when one eye is closed.

Loss of side vision from a stroke usually occurs suddenly but may be noticed only later on. Because the right side of the brain controls the left half of the visual field of each eye and vice versa, a person with a stroke on one side of the brain may notice that he or she can only see half of objects on the other side of the vision. These visual field defects often affect both eyes equally.

Vision problems are only some of the symptoms of stroke. In many strokes patients experience weakness, numbness, or tingling in other parts of the body.

Examination Findings: What the Doctor Looks for · In evaluating patients with stroke and double vision, the eye doctor examines the eye movements, often measuring the amount of eye misalignment when the patient looks in different directions. If a stroke is suspected, the eye doctor will check the side vision, either by asking the patient to say, using only his or her side vision, how many fingers the doctor is holding up, or by performing computerized visual field testing.

What You Can Do · The best treatment for stroke is prevention. Maintaining a healthy lifestyle, controlling your blood pressure, and controlling your blood sugar if you are diabetic are important. If you smoke, talk to your doctor about the risk of stroke posed by tobacco use and about ways to stop smoking.

When to Call the Doctor · If you experience double vision, a sudden loss of side vision, or new weakness, numbness, or tingling in other parts of your body, go to the nearest emergency room immediately. Some stroke treatments are only available if you can be treated within the first few hours.

Treatment · Treatment for the visual complications of stroke is indicated once your overall medical condition is stable. Patients with recent stroke often need to be hospitalized for several days, because controlling blood pressure to help maximize blood flow to the brain is a key component of therapy. New treatments to help minimize brain injury after stroke are currently being evaluated.

Once you are medically stable, specific therapy for vision problems may be undertaken. In some patients with cranial nerve palsies causing double vision, special glasses with prisms may help to better align the images from the two eyes so that the brain sees objects as single. In other cases, eye muscle surgery may relieve double vision by helping to restore eye movement and alignment. In patients with side vision defects, a consultation with a vision rehabilitation specialist may be helpful to maximize the remaining vision.

Prognosis: Will I See Better? · In most cases double vision from stroke can be treated successfully. If eye muscle surgery is indicated, more than one surgery may be necessary over time, since there is no way to exactly predict eye alignment after eye muscle surgery. Currently no specific therapy to restore damaged peripheral vision exists. However, vision rehabilitation specialists are often successful in helping patients learn to use their remaining vision to resume many of their daily activities, including reading, housework, and hobbies.

http://www.eyemdlink.com/Condition.asp?ConditionID=427
www.nanosweb.org/patient_info/brochures/

Human Immunodeficiency Virus

KELLY WALTON MUIR, M.D.

What Is It? · Human immunodeficiency virus (HIV) is the virus that causes Acquired Immune Deficiency Syndrome, or AIDS. HIV is carried in blood and bodily fluids and is transmitted whenever these fluids are transmitted, such as during sex, blood transfusions, the sharing of dirty needles, and childbirth. Tests are available to screen pregnant women and donated blood for HIV, so the primary modes of transmission currently are sex and intravenous drug abuse accompanied by the sharing of dirty needles. The virus attacks the body's immune system and leaves the victim vulnerable to multiple infections. AIDS is defined by the presence of opportunistic infections in a person infected by HIV, or by severe damage to the immune system from HIV without opportunistic infection. Up to 75% of patients with AIDS will experience eye complications but may be asymptomatic in many cases.

Symptoms: What You May Experience · HIV can live in the body for many years before it causes symptoms. Unexplained weight loss, fatigue, and repeated skin infections suggest the possibility of AIDS. Eye complications from HIV may cause decreased vision or eye pain.

Examination Findings: What the Doctor Looks for · Your eye doctor will look for signs of eye infection, inflammation, tumor, or damage to the retinal blood vessels from HIV.

What You Can Do · AIDS is a preventable disease. To avoid exposing your body to HIV, treat all blood and bodily fluids as if they are infected.

When to Call the Doctor · If you experience recurrent infections or unexplained weight loss, you should talk to your primary care doctor about HIV. If you have HIV, you should have a complete eye exam annually. Patients with HIV who notice eye pain, redness, or blurry vision should contact their eye doctor.

Treatment · There are many new medications available to treat HIV, but still no cure exists. Your ophthalmologist can recommend treatment options for the eye complications of HIV and AIDS.

Prognosis: Will I See Better? · With new anti-HIV medications, patients who have the disease are living longer and experiencing fewer complications. Despite the best care, however, some patients with HIV suffer from permanent visual loss.

http://www.cdc.gov/hiv/dhap.htm http://www.aegis.org/

16 · Cosmetic Eyelid Surgery

JULIE A. WOODWARD, M.D.

As time passes, our eyelids become droopy with the natural aging process. The entire forehead and eyebrows can also droop, which adds to the droopy appearance of the eyelids. Tissues that once were firm become softer, allowing the natural fat surrounding the eyeballs to herniate, or bulge forward, thus creating "bags" under the eyes. These bags cast shadows on the thin, bony, lower rim of the orbit, emphasizing dark circles under the eyes.

There are two types of wrinkles that affect the face and eyes. Dynamic wrinkles occur when we make facial expressions. An example of dynamic wrinkles is the wrinkles in the crow's feet areas (at the outer corner of the eyes) that increase when we smile. These dynamic wrinkles are often caused by thickening of some of the eyelid and facial muscles surrounding the eyes that occurs with age. Thickened muscles in the lower eyelids look like little bags beneath the eyelashes, while thickened muscles in the forehead emphasize the vertical frown lines between the eyebrows. The wrinkles that are present when the face is still are called static wrinkles, which are caused by the breakdown of skin collagen from sun damage.

While some tissues, such as the eyelid muscles, become thickened with age, other tissues become thinned. The skin overlying the bony rim of the orbit surrounding each eye becomes thin, which adds to the appearance of dark circles under the eyes. Beneath this area is another area of skin thinning along a ligament in the cheek. This area delineates a second "bag," which lies between the lower eyelid and the cheek and is called a festoon.

Oculoplastic surgery is a subspeciality field of ophthalmology that is concerned with both cosmetic and functional aspects of the eyes and surrounding facial structures. The following procedures are examples of typical cosmetic oculoplastic surgeries designed to improve the effects of aging on the eyelids.

Upper Eyelid Blepharoplasty · Blepharoplasty is the medical term for eyelid lift. The surgeon may use various instruments to perform blepharoplasty surgery, including a steel blade, a laser, or a heated cautery instrument. The laser and the cautery are particularly useful for decreasing bleeding during the procedure. Regardless of the technique used, the result is similar. This outpatient surgery is typically performed in the operating room or minor operating room with sedation and locally injected numbing medication.

An upper eyelid blepharoplasty is a procedure to lift the tissues in the upper eyelid. First, an incision is made in the upper eyelid crease, where it will remain hidden afterward. The amount of drooping skin, muscle, and herniated fat in the upper eyelid is carefully measured by the ophthalmologist during surgery to determine how much can be removed above the eyelid crease, while ensuring that the patient can still comfortably close his or her eyes after surgery. The wound is stitched closed at the end of the procedure, and an antibiotic ointment is placed on the incision for about 7–10 days. The stitches are usually removed in the office one week after surgery.

Brow Lift · If the eyebrows sag downward because of age and gravity, they can be lifted in a surgery called a brow, or forehead, lift. This surgery can be combined with an upper eyelid blepharoplasty. There are two common methods for operating on sagging brows. In a direct brow lift, an incision is made along the top edge of each eyebrow and excess skin and muscle are removed. The eyebrows are then lifted when the incisions are closed with stitches. In an endoscopic brow lift, incisions are made in the hairline, where the scars will be less noticeable. A tiny camera on the end of a lighted wand is inserted into the hairline incisions and used to place stitches that lift the eyebrows upward.

Lower Eyelid Blepharoplasty · Lower eyelid blepharoplasty is a procedure to remove bulging fat bags under the lower eyelids. Some surgeons perform transcutaneous blepharoplasty by removing the fat bags through the skin beneath the eyelashes. This requires skin stitches for the incision at the end of the procedure. Other surgeons approach the fat through the inside of the lower eyelid in a method called transconjunctival blepharoplasty, which does not require skin stitches.

Removing the lower eyelid fat bags can result in loose skin in this area in some patients. There are two commonly used techniques to tighten this loose skin during a lower eyelid blepharoplasty. In the first technique, typically used in transcutaneous blepharoplasty, the loose skin can be cut out just beneath the skin incision, taking care not to remove so much skin that the lower eyelid is pulled down out of position. The second technique to tighten the loose skin is laser skin resurfacing. A specialized laser vaporizes the top layer of skin and causes the loose skin to contract. This technique can be used to minimize wrinkles on the entire face. As the skin heals after the laser resurfacing, the patient may be instructed to cleanse and moisturize the skin frequently and avoid makeup for at least 10 days following the procedure. Also, the resurfaced skin may remain slightly pink for up to 4–6 months after laser treatment, which may require camouflage makeup.

Botulinum Toxin (Botox) · Botulinum toxin, or Botox, is a medication injected to paralyze muscles. Botulinum toxin injection is a popular method of treating dynamic wrinkles when the medication is injected into certain muscles of the face. Typically botulinum toxin is injected with a tiny needle into the facial muscles in the forehead and surrounding the eyes during an office visit. The medication usually requires several days to take effect and lasts for 3–4 months, after which the injections can be repeated.

http://www.asoprs.org/Pages/blepharoplasty.html
http://www.fda.gov/fdac/features/2002/402_botox.html

17 · Living with Visual Impairment

RENEE HALBERG, MSW, LCSW

Understanding Feelings · Vision loss happens to people of all ages. With vision loss, it is normal to experience feelings of sadness, anger, frustration, guilt, or fear. It is also common to feel a loss of independence and self-esteem and to be concerned about becoming a burden to loved ones. Family members also react to vision loss in different ways: denial, acceptance, withdrawal, overprotection, or avoidance. Often it is not easy to admit to having these feelings. Please try to remember that these feelings are not right or wrong.

People who lose some or all of their vision may enter a period of grieving. How you feel is typically influenced by the degree and stability of your vision loss, your age, what is learned from your family, your cultural and religious beliefs, and the type of support system you have.

Ways to Help · For caregivers of people with vision loss, it is important to be a good listener and to encourage independence and social interaction. Resist the urge to be overly sympathetic or protective. It is also helpful for caregivers to understand what their loved one can see and do. Remember that all people with vision loss do not see the same.

If you have vision loss, it may be difficult to talk about how your vision loss affects your loved ones. You may feel concerned that you are hurting the feelings of your caregivers or other family members. However, sharing information with your family and friends about how your vision loss affects your everyday life can make it easier for others to offer help. Try to have important conversations when all parties are calm; openly discussing how vision loss affects all of your lives can help you feel closer to loved ones. When friends and family are not enough, consider attending a support group. There are numerous support groups across the United States for people with vision loss from all sorts of eye diseases. Joining a support group can help you to learn from others, feel connected to those who understand what you are experiencing, and lessen feelings of anxiety and aloneness. Support groups can also help you find solutions and gain new perspectives on living with vision loss. In this Internet age, it is easier than ever to contact other patients with eye diseases and to share insights and experiences through support groups' web sites.

If you or a loved one lives with vision loss, make the effort to explore available community resources. Virtually every county or city has government-sponsored services, most of which are free of charge, for people with visual impairment. These services can include special libraries with large-print or recorded books, or help in finding and purchasing low-vision aids. Tax benefits for people with impaired vision also exist.

When to Ask for Professional Help · A low-vision specialist is a professional trained to help people with impaired vision to perform their daily activities. If you visit a low-vision specialist in your community, he or she will demonstrate different visual aids and help you decide which ones will help you. These aids can include magnifiers (in glasses, hand-held, on a stand, or electronic), computerized reading devices, and other tools to help you perform your daily tasks. Not all these aids may suit your needs, but exploring them is a good first step to learning to make the most of your vision.

Some low-vision specialists are experts in visual rehabilitation. These professionals will often come to your home to help you set up a user-friendly environment that serves your visual needs, and they can help you learn special techniques to perform your daily activities more effectively and with less frustration.

It is not unusual to experience high and low moods when dealing with vision loss. When the low periods interfere with your ability to function and just won't go away, you may be suffering from depression, a serious, common illness. Other signs of depression are a loss of interest in pleasurable activities, significant weight loss or gain, inability to sleep or sleeping too much, social withdrawal, frequent crying spells, irritability, anxiety, feelings of hopelessness and helplessness, and difficulty concentrating. If you have depression, it is essential to get professional help from a skilled and licensed professional. You can ask your primary care physician for a referral to a licensed clinical social worker, psychologist, psychiatric nurse, or psychiatrist. For family members, it is a life-threatening emergency if a loved one expresses suicidal thoughts and plans. Call 911 and have the person taken to the nearest hospital for assessment and treatment.

Creative Ways to Deal with Stress · We need to take care of ourselves in order to live fulfilling lives. Think about what brings you joy, encourages laughter, or gives you a sense of peace. Try taking a walk, signing up for a dance or yoga class, learning to meditate, listening to your favorite music, or using aromatherapy. Perhaps you would like to plant flowers and herbs, sculpt with clay, or record your life story on tape for your family. Spend time with other people who have a positive attitude and a sense of humor, and you will realize that you are not alone as you live with visual impairment.

http://www.preventblindness.org/ http://www.afb.org/
www.aerbvi.org/ http://www.lighthouse.org/ http://www.loc.gov/nls/

Appendix: Major Clinical Trials

JENNIFER S. WEIZER, M.D.

Herpetic Eye Disease Study

· *Main Questions Tested*: How is infectious keratitis that is caused by the herpes simplex virus best treated?

· *Main Findings*: In certain situations, steroid eye drops, antiviral eye drops, and oral antiviral medication can help treat herpes simplex keratitis successfully.

· *Comments*: Appropriate treatment depends on the exact location and type of the herpes simplex virus infection.

Diabetic Retinopathy Study

· *Main Questions Tested*: Does retinal laser treatment help prevent visual loss from diabetic retinopathy?

· *Main Findings*: Retinal laser treatment reduced severe visual loss from diabetic retinopathy by 50%.

· *Comments*: Only certain severe forms of diabetic retinopathy were considered appropriate for laser treatment.

Early Treatment of Diabetic Retinopathy Study

· *Main Questions Tested*: When should retinal laser treatment be performed for diabetic retinopathy? Does retinal laser treatment help treat diabetic macular edema? Does taking aspirin affect diabetic retinopathy?

· *Main Findings*: Certain severe forms of diabetic retinopathy are considered appropriate for laser treatment. Retinal laser treatment of diabetic macular edema reduces the risk of moderate vision loss by 50%. Aspirin does not affect diabetic retinopathy.

Diabetic Retinopathy Vitrectomy Study

· *Main Questions Tested*: Does vitrectomy surgery help severe cases of diabetic retinopathy?

· *Main Findings*: In certain severe cases of diabetic retinopathy, vitrectomy surgery can be beneficial.

· *Comments*: Whether vitrectomy surgery is appropriate depends on the exact type and severity of the diabetic retinopathy.

Endophthalmitis Vitrectomy Study

· *Main Questions Tested*: Which is better for treating endophthalmitis after cataract surgery—injection of antibiotics into the eyeball or vitrectomy surgery?

· *Main Findings*: For endophthalmitis with vision of hand motion or better, injection of antibiotics in the eyeball is the best treatment. For endophthalmitis with vision worse than hand motion, vitrectomy surgery is the best treatment.

· *Comments*: Intravenous antibiotics did not help treat endophthalmitis.

Macular Photocoagulation Study

· *Main Questions Tested*: Does laser treatment help treat abnormal blood vessels that grow in the wet form of age-related macular degeneration?

· *Main Findings*: Certain forms of abnormal blood vessels benefited from laser treatment.

· *Comments*: The success of the laser treatment depended on the exact type, size, and location of the abnormal blood vessels.

Treatment of Age-Related Macular Degeneration with Photodynamic Therapy Study

· *Main Questions Tested*: Does photodynamic therapy help treat abnormal blood vessels that grow in certain types of wet age-related macular generation?

· *Main Findings*: Photodynamic therapy can reduce the risk of vision loss in certain types of wet age-related macular degeneration.

· *Comments*: The success of the photodynamic therapy depended on the exact type, size, and location of the abnormal blood vessels.

Eye Disease Case-Control Study

· *Main Questions Tested*: Do dietary carotenoids and vitamins A, C, and E help reduce the risk of developing wet age-related macular degeneration?

· *Main Findings*: Eating more carotenoids, particularly lutein and zeaxanthin, was associated with lower risk of wet age-related macular degeneration. Vitamins A, C, and E were not definitely found to reduce the risk of wet age-related macular degeneration.

· *Comments*: Lutein and zeaxanthin are most commonly found in dark green, leafy vegetables.

Age-Related Eye Disease Study

· *Main Questions Tested*: Do certain high-dose vitamins and minerals help slow the progression of age-related macular degeneration?

· *Main Findings*: Certain high doses of vitamins C and E, beta-carotene, zinc, and copper can slow the progression of certain forms of age-related macular degeneration.

· *Comments*: Smokers should not take beta-carotene. Consult your eye doctor about whether these vitamins would benefit your type of macular degeneration. Consult your primary medical doctor about whether these high-dose vitamins are safe for you to take.

Central Vein Occlusion Study

· *Main Questions Tested*: What is the natural course of central retinal vein occlusion? Does laser treatment help treat central retinal vein occlusion?

· *Main Findings*: Vision tended to stay fairly stable over time after a central retinal vein occlusion occurred, although some eyes had worsened vision. Laser treatment can help to prevent further complications in certain types of central retinal vein occlusion.

Branch Vein Occlusion Study

· *Main Questions Tested*: Does laser treatment help treat branch retinal vein occlusion?

· *Main Findings*: Laser treatment can help prevent further complications in certain types of branch retinal vein occlusion.

· *Comments*: The type of laser and the success of laser treatment depended on the type and severity of the branch retinal vein occlusion.

Standard Care vs. Corticosteroid for Retinal Vein Occlusion Study
· *Main Questions Tested*: Does steroid medication injected in the eyeball help treat retinal vein occlusion?
· *Comments*: Currently in progress.

Advanced Glaucoma Intervention Study
· *Main Questions Tested*: Which surgical treatment should be performed first when treating primary open angle glaucoma — laser treatment or trabeculectomy?
· *Main Findings*: In black patients, laser treatment performed first may be more beneficial in preventing vision loss. In white patients, trabeculectomy performed first may be more beneficial.
· *Comments*: The appropriate surgical treatment depends mostly on each patient's particular case.

Collaborative Initial Glaucoma Treatment Study
· *Main Questions Tested*: Should newly diagnosed glaucoma patients be treated first with pressure-lowering eye drops or trabeculectomy surgery?
· *Main Findings*: Patients did equally well over time with either eye drops or trabeculectomy surgery.
· *Comments*: Because using eye drops for glaucoma is generally lower risk than performing trabeculectomy surgery, many eye doctors will begin treatment with eye drops.

Early Manifest Glaucoma Trial
· *Main Questions Tested*: Should patients with early glaucoma receive treatment to lower their eye pressure or be monitored without treatment?
· *Main Findings*: Treating early glaucoma patients with eye drops or laser to lower eye pressure slowed the progression of glaucoma damage.

Ocular Hypertension Treatment Study
· *Main Questions Tested*: Should patients with high eye pressure

but no obvious glaucoma damage receive treatment to lower eye pressure?

· *Main Findings*: Treating patients with high eye pressure but no glaucoma damage reduced the risk of developing glaucoma damage in the future by 50%.

· *Comments*: The decision whether to treat a patient with high eye pressure depends on many other factors as well and is based on each patient's particular case.

Normal Tension Glaucoma Study

· *Main Questions Tested*: In glaucoma patients whose eye pressure is not high, does lowering the eye pressure help treat the glaucoma?

· *Main Findings*: Lowering eye pressure by 30% with treatment reduces the progression of glaucoma even if the starting eye pressure was not high.

Optic Neuritis Treatment Trial

· *Main Questions Tested*: Does steroid medication help treat optic neuritis?

· *Main Findings*: Intravenous steroid medication can speed recovery from optic neuritis. Oral steroid medication alone does not help treat optic neuritis.

· *Comments*: Intravenous steroid medication does not affect how much vision is ultimately restored after an episode of optic neuritis.

Cryotherapy for Retinopathy of Prematurity

· *Main Questions Tested*: Does cryotherapy help treat retinopathy of prematurity?

· *Main Findings*: In certain severe cases of retinopathy of prematurity, cryotherapy can reduce the risk of vision loss by 40%.

· *Comments*: Cryotherapy is now often replaced by laser therapy.

http://www.nei.nih.gov/neitrials/all-alpha.aspx

Glossary

abscess collection of pus

accommodation a slight change in the shape of the natural lens that allows one to see nearby objects

achromatopsia a retinal disease in which no colors are seen

Acquired Immune Deficiency Syndrome (AIDS) an infectious disease that weakens the body's immune system

acute hydrops a painful episode of corneal swelling usually seen in keratoconus

"after cataract" (posterior capsular opacity) a film that forms behind a lens implant

age-related macular degeneration a disease of older people that affects the center of the retina (macula)

amblyopia (lazy eye) decreased vision in one or both eyes that is caused by disruption of normal visual development from a variety of causes

anterior chamber the space inside the eyeball between the cornea and the front of the iris

aqueous humor the clear fluid that fills the anterior chamber of the eye

astigmatism an irregular curvature of the surface of the cornea

atrophy permanent loss of a part of the body

autoimmune involving a malfunction of the body's immune system

basal cell carcinoma a type of skin cancer

benign noncancerous

black eye (orbital ecchymosis) a collection of fluid and blood in the tissues around the eye

blepharitis inflammation of the eyelid margins

blepharoplasty surgery to lift the eyelids

blepharospasm uncontrolled twitching of the muscles in the eyelids and around the eyes

blue-yellow color deficiency an inherited difficulty in distinguishing between blue and yellow colors

botulinum toxin (Botox) a medicine injected into the muscles to paralyze them

brow lift surgery to lift the eyebrows

Bruch's membrane a layer of tis-

sue that separates the retina
and retinal pigment epithelium
from the choroid

capsular bag the natural bag that
holds a lens or lens implant in
place in the pupil of the eye

carcinoma a type of cancer

cataract a clouding of the normally clear lens inside the eye

cellophane retinopathy (epiretinal
membrane, macular pucker,
preretinal gliosis) a thin sheet
of abnormal scar tissue that
grows over the retina

central nervous system the brain,
the spinal cord, and their
nerves

central retinal artery the blood
vessel that supplies most of the
retina

central retinal vein the blood
vessel that drains most of the
retina

central serous chorioretinopathy
a disease in which fluid collects
under the macula

cerebrospinal fluid (CSF) fluid
that surrounds the brain, spinal
cord, and optic nerves

chalazion a nodule of inflammation that forms a bump in the
eyelid

choroid a blood vessel layer
located between the retina and
sclera

choroidal neovascularization
(CNV) a patch of abnormal
blood vessels and scar tissue
that grows under the retina

ciliary body the part of the eyeball
that produces aqueous humor

colorblindness a deficiency in the
way color is seen

computed tomography (CT scan)
a specialized x-ray technique

cone a type of photoreceptor
that processes colors and finely
detailed images

congenital present at birth

conjunctiva the outer, clear tissue
layer that covers the white part
of the eyeball

conjunctivitis (pink eye) inflammation of the conjunctiva

cornea the clear, round, central window in the front of the
eyeball overlying the pupil,
through which light travels to
enter the eye

corneal abrasion a scratch on the
cornea

corneal transplant a surgical procedure to replace a diseased
cornea with a healthy donor
cornea

corneal ulcer a deep infection in
the cornea

cranial nerve one of twelve specialized nerves from the brain
that control different parts of
the eye, head, neck, and chest

cryotherapy freezing treatment

cystoid macular edema a disease
in which fluid leaks into the

macula and collects to form cysts

dacryocystitis infection of the tear drainage system

dacryocystorhinostomy (DCR) a surgical procedure to repair a blocked tear drainage system

diabetes mellitus a disease of abnormal blood sugar regulation

diabetic macular edema swelling in the central retina caused by diabetes

diabetic retinopathy a retinal disease caused by diabetes

diplopia double vision

dislocated lens a lens or lens implant that moves out of the capsular bag; or a lens or lens implant that moves out of the proper position along with the capsular bag

drusen aging deposits located under the retina

dry eye syndrome an abnormality of the tear film that lubricates the surface of the eye

dynamic wrinkles wrinkles that occur with facial expressions

ectropion an outward turning of the eyelid margin away from the eyeball

edema swelling

electroretinogram a special electrical test used mainly to examine retinal function

endophthalmitis a severe infection inside the eyeball

entropion an inward turning of the eyelid margin toward the eyeball

epiretinal membrane (cellophane retinopathy, macular pucker, preretinal gliosis) a thin sheet of abnormal scar tissue that grows over the retina

episclera the connective tissue layer between the conjunctiva and the sclera

episcleritis inflammation of the episclera

esotropia misalignment of an eye, in toward the nose

exotropia misalignment of an eye, out toward the ear on the same side

eyelid margin the edge of the eyelid where eyelashes grow

eye M.D. (ophthalmologist) a medical doctor trained to perform eye surgery who examines and treats all eye conditions

eye socket (orbit) the cavity in the head in which the eyeball sits

festoon a lower bag that forms between the lower eyelid and the cheek with aging

floater a spot that appears to drift in one's visual field, usually because of an opacity in the vitreous cavity

fluorescein angiogram a special photographic dye test used to examine the retina

focal laser a laser technique used mainly to treat macular edema

fusion the ability of the brain to process and blend images coming from both eyes

giant cell arteritis (temporal arteritis) an inflammatory disease of blood vessels

glaucoma a disease of the optic nerve, often associated with high eye pressure

Graves disease an autoimmune disorder that is the most common cause of hyperthyroidism

grid laser a laser technique used mainly to treat macular edema

hemoglobin A1C a blood test that measures the average blood sugar level over the previous three months

herniate to bulge or pouch forward

high-order aberrations optical imperfections that can distort the quality of vision and are not correctable by glasses or contact lenses

hordeolum (stye) a nodule of inflammation and infection that forms a bump in the eyelid

human immunodeficiency virus (HIV) the virus that causes Acquired Immune Deficiency Syndrome (AIDS)

hyperopia farsightedness

hypertension high blood pressure

hypertensive retinopathy a retinal disease caused by high blood pressure

hyperthyroidism overactivity of the thyroid gland

hypertropia misalignment of an eye upward

hyphema blood in the anterior chamber of the eye

hypotony low eye pressure

hypotropia misalignment of an eye downward

intraocular foreign body an object inside the eyeball that is not naturally found there

iris the colored, circular part of the eye that surrounds the pupil

keratitis inflammation of the cornea

keratoconus a condition in which the cornea is abnormally steep and cone-shaped

laceration a wound or tear

lacrimal gland an orbital structure responsible for producing tears

LASEK (laser epithelial keratomileusis) a type of refractive surgery designed to improve one's unaided vision

laser retinopexy a laser technique used mainly to "tack down" the retina surrounding a retinal tear

laser skin resurfacing a technique

in which a specialized laser is used to tighten the skin

laser trabeculoplasty a laser technique used mainly to treat certain types of glaucoma

LASIK (laser-assisted in situ keratomileusis) a type of refractive surgery designed to improve one's unaided vision

lens the lentil-shaped part of the eye behind the pupil that helps to focus light

leukocoria a white pupil

limbus the outer edge of the cornea

lumbar puncture (spinal tap) a test to withdraw the fluid that surrounds the spinal cord and brain

macula the central area of the retina, responsible for central vision

macular edema swelling in the central retina

macular hole a hole in the central retina

macular ischemia reduced blood flow to the macula

macular pucker (cellophane retinopathy, epiretinal membrane, preretinal gliosis) a thin sheet of abnormal scar tissue that grows over the retina

macular translocation a surgical technique used mainly for certain types of age-related macular degeneration

magnetic resonance imaging (MRI scan) a specialized x-ray technique

malignant cancerous

melanoma a cancer of pigment-containing cells in the skin or eye

meninges the three layers of tissue that surround the optic nerve and brain

metastatic a cancer that has spread from another part of the body

migraine an attack of neurologic or mood disturbance which often, but not always, includes headache

multiple sclerosis (MS) a disease of the brain and spinal cord in which the body attacks its own central nervous system

myopia nearsightedness

neovascular glaucoma glaucoma caused by growth of abnormal new blood vessels in the drain of the eye

neovascularization growth of abnormal new blood vessels

neuro-ophthalmologist an eye M.D. who specializes in the optic nerves and the eye's connections to the brain

nevus a mole or pigmented lesion found on the skin or in the eye

occipital lobe the part of the brain located at the back of the head where vision is processed

ocular prosthesis an artificial eyeball that does not see

ocularist a professional who specializes in making ocular prostheses

oculoplastic surgery a subspeciality field of ophthalmology that is concerned with cosmetic and functional aspects of the tissues surrounding the eyeballs

open globe a condition in which there is a full-thickness wound to the wall of the eyeball

ophthalmologist (eye M.D.) a medical doctor trained to perform eye surgery who examines and treats all eye conditions

opportunistic infection an infection that attacks weak, but not healthy, immune systems

optic canal a passageway through which nerves and blood vessels travel between the eye and the brain

optic chiasm an area in the brain where the optic nerves are joined

optic nerve the part of the eye that carries visual information from the eyeball to the brain

optic nerve sheath decompression a surgical procedure to relieve pressure on the optic nerve from its surrounding fluid

optic neuritis inflammation of the optic nerve

optic neuropathy abnormal function of the optic nerve

optic radiations nerve fibers in the brain that carry information from the optic tracts to the visual cortex

optic tract a structure in the brain that carries information from the optic chiasm to the optic radiations

optical coherence tomogram (OCT) a special non-x-ray photographic test used to examine the macula

optician an eye care professional who fits and dispenses corrective eyewear

optometrist an eye care professional who examines the eye, prescribes glasses and contact lenses, and medically treats certain eye conditions

ora serrata the part of the eyeball just behind the ciliary body where the retina ends

orbit (eye socket) the cavity in the head in which the eyeball sits

orbital blow-out fracture a break in one or more of the bones that make up the orbit and surround the eyeball

orbital cellulitis an infection in the orbit

orbital ecchymosis (black eye) a collection of fluid and blood in the tissues around the eye

orbital septum a thin layer of

tissue behind the eyelids that helps prevent eyelid infections from reaching the orbit

pachymetry a technique used to measure the thickness of the cornea

panretinal laser photocoagulation (PRP) a laser technique used mainly to treat retinal neovascularization

papilledema swelling of the optic nerves caused by increased cerebrospinal fluid pressure around the brain

pars planitis inflammation in the front and middle parts of the eyeball

peripheral iridectomy a surgical or laser technique in which a tiny hole is made in the iris to prevent or treat certain types of glaucoma

phacoemulsification a method of surgically removing a cataract using ultrasound

photodynamic therapy (PDT) a special laser treatment used to treat certain types of wet age-related macular degeneration

photoreceptor a specialized cell in the retina that converts light images into electrical signals

pink eye (conjunctivitis) inflammation of the conjunctiva

pneumatic retinopexy a special technique involving cryo-therapy and bubble injections to treat certain retinal detachments

polycarbonate an impact-resistant material used in the lenses of eyeglasses

posterior capsular opacity ("after cataract") a film that forms behind a lens implant

posterior chamber the space inside the eyeball between the back of the iris and the front of the vitreous gel

posterior vitreous detachment separation of the vitreous gel from the inner surface of the retina

preretinal gliosis (cellophane retinopathy, epiretinal membrane, macular pucker) a thin sheet of abnormal scar tissue that grows over the retina

presbyopia decreased ability to see near objects that occurs with aging

preseptal cellulitis infection of the eyelids and surrounding skin and soft tissues

PRK (photorefractive keratectomy) a type of refractive surgery designed to improve one's unaided vision

pseudotumor cerebri a disease in which cerebrospinal fluid pressure is elevated without a known cause

ptosis a drooping upper eyelid

pupil the dark, round space in the center of the iris

radial keratotomy (RK) an early refractive surgery technique designed to improve one's unaided level of vision

red-green color deficiency an inherited difficulty in distinguishing between red and green colors

refract to bend light

refraction testing a person's eyes for glasses

refractive surgery a group of surgical techniques designed to improve one's unaided level of vision

retina a thin layer of complex nerve tissue that lines the inside back wall of the eyeball

retinal artery occlusion blockage of an artery that supplies blood to the retina

retinal break a hole or tear in the retina

retinal detachment an abnormal separation of the retina from the inner wall of the eyeball

retinal vein occlusion blockage of a vein that drains blood from the retina

retinitis pigmentosa a group of inherited retinal degenerative diseases

retinoblastoma a cancer of primitive retinal cells that grows inside the eyeball

rod a type of photoreceptor that processes dark and light images

sclera the white, outer layer of the eyeball

scleral buckling a surgical technique to treat retinal detachments

scleritis inflammation of the sclera

sebaceous cell carcinoma a rare cancer arising from eyelid oil glands

silicone oil a special material used to fill the eyeball after certain vitrectomy surgeries

slit lamp an illuminating microscope to examine the front part of the eye

spinal tap (lumbar puncture) a test to withdraw the fluid that surrounds the spinal cord and brain

squamous cell carcinoma a type of skin cancer

static wrinkles wrinkles that are present when the face is still

stereopsis depth perception

steroid a type of anti-inflammatory medication

strabismus misalignment of one or both eyes

stroke a disease in which brain tissue is damaged by lack of blood supply

stye (hordeolum) a nodule of inflammation and infection that forms a bump in the eyelid

subconjunctival hemorrhage a collection of blood that accumulates under the conjunctiva

subluxed lens a lens or lens implant that shifts but stays within the capsular bag

tarsorrhaphy a surgical procedure to attach the eyelids together

temporal arteritis (giant cell arteritis) an inflammatory disease of blood vessels

thyroid eye disease a set of eye problems typically associated with thyroid disease

toric a type of contact lens or lens implant that corrects astigmatism

trabeculectomy a type of glaucoma surgery

uveal tract the pigmented portion of the eyeball that includes the iris, ciliary body, and choroid

uveitis inflammation of the uveal tract inside the eyeball

verteporfin (Visudyne) a special dye used in photodynamic therapy

viral retinitis inflammation of the retina caused by a virus

virus an organism that lives by infecting other living cells

vision rehabilitation specialist a professional who helps people with impaired vision maximize their vision so that they can perform daily activities

visual acuity a person's level of vision

visual cortex the area of the brain at the back of the head where vision is processed

visual field peripheral or side vision

Visudyne (verteporfin) a special dye used in photodynamic therapy

vitrectomy a surgical procedure to remove the vitreous from the vitreous cavity in the back of the eyeball

vitreous the natural gel that fills the back of the eyeball

vitreous cavity the space in the eyeball that contains the vitreous

wavefront a type of technology used to customize refractive surgery for each individual patient

x-linked an inheritance pattern in which mothers pass a gene to their children but only their sons usually show the effect of the gene

zonule a fiber that holds the capsular bag and lens in position

Authors' Affiliations

NATALIE A. AFSHARI, M.D. · Duke University Eye Center, Durham, N.C.

ROSANNA P. BAHADUR, M.D. · Private practice, Charlotte, N.C.

SRILAXMI BEARELLY, M.D. · Duke University Eye Center, Durham, N.C.

SCOTT BLACKMON, M.D. · Duke University Eye Center, Durham, N.C.

ALAN N. CARLSON, M.D. · Duke University Eye Center, Durham, N.C.

PRATAP CHALLA, M.D. · Duke University Eye Center, Durham, N.C.

HELEN CHANDLER, O.D. · Duke University Eye Center, Durham, N.C.

RAVI CHANDRASHEKHAR, M.D., MSEE · Wilson Regional Medical
Center, Johnson City, N.Y.

DAVID A. CHESNUTT, M.D. · Duke University Eye Center, Durham, N.C.

CLAUDIA S. COHEN, M.D. · Private practice, Durham, N.C.

MICHAEL J. COONEY, M.D. · Duke University Eye Center, Durham, N.C.

THOMAS J. CUMMINGS, M.D. · Department of Pathology, Duke
University Medical Center, Durham, N.C.

VINCENT A. DERAMO, M.D. · Private practice, Great Neck, N.Y.

LAURA ENYEDI, M.D. · Duke University Eye Center, Durham, N.C.

SHARON FEKRAT, M.D. · Duke University Eye Center, Durham, N.C.

HERB GREENMAN, M.D. · Private practice, Charlotte, N.C.

RENEE HALBERG, MSW, LCSW · Duke University Eye Center,
Durham, N.C.

DEREK HESS, M.D. · Private practice, St. Petersburg, Fla.

PAUL KANG, M.D. · Private practice, Chevy Chase, Md.

PAUL KURZ, M.D. · Private practice, Saginaw, Mich.

PAUL P. LEE, M.D., J.D. · Duke University Eye Center, Durham, N.C.

BROOKS W. MCCUEN II, M.D. · Duke University Eye Center,
Durham, N.C.

PRIYATHAM S. METTU, M.D. · Duke University Eye Center, Durham, N.C.

JOHN J. MICHON, M.D. · Duke University Eye Center, Durham, N.C.

PRITHVI MRUTHYUNJAYA, M.D. · Duke University Eye Center, Durham, N.C.

KELLY WALTON MUIR, M.D. · Duke University Eye Center, Durham, N.C.

KENNETH NEUFELD, M.D. · Private practice, Atlanta

MILA OH, M.D. · Department of Ophthalmology, McGill University, Montreal

SHERMAN W. REEVES, M.D., MPH · Duke University Eye Center, Durham, N.C.

PAUL S. RISKE, M.D. · Private practice, Raleigh, N.C.

DIANNA L. SELDOMRIDGE, M.D., MBA · Department of Ophthalmology, Rush University Medical Center, Chicago

TERRY SEMCHYSHYN, M.D. · Duke University Eye Center, Durham, N.C.

INDER PAUL SINGH, M.D. · Private practice, Racine, Wis.

JULIA SONG, M.D. · Private practice, San Diego

CYNTHIA A. TOTH, M.D. · Duke University Eye Center, Durham, N.C.

JENNIFER SOMERS WEIZER, M.D. · Kellogg Eye Center, University of Michigan, Ann Arbor

KATRINA P. WINTER, M.D. · Duke University Eye Center, Durham, N.C.

JULIE A. WOODWARD, M.D. · Duke University Eye Center, Durham, N.C.

DAVID YEH, M.D. · Cullen Eye Institute, Baylor College of Medicine, Houston

CAROL J. ZIEL, M.D. · Duke University Eye Center, Durham, N.C.

Index

Page numbers in *italics* refer to illustrations.

SHARON FEKRAT, M.D., FACS,

is a practicing vitreoretinal surgeon and

associate professor in the Department of

Ophthalmology, Duke University. She is

president-elect of the North Carolina Society

of Eye Physicians and Surgeons.

JENNIFER S. WEIZER, M.D.,

is a clinical assistant professor at the Kellogg

Eye Center, University of Michigan.

Library of Congress Cataloging-in-Publication Data

All about your eyes / Sharon Fekrat and
Jennifer S. Weizer, eds. ; illustrations
by Stanley M. Coffman.
p. cm.
Includes bibliographical references and index.
ISBN 0-8223-3660-x (cloth : alk. paper)
ISBN 0-8223-3699-5 (pbk. : alk. paper)
1. Eye—Diseases. 2. Ophthalmology.
I. Fekrat, Sharon.
II. Weizer, Jennifer S.
RE46.A44 2006
617.7—dc22   2005025674